My
Breast

Joyce Wadler is a former New York correspondent of the *Washington Post*. At the time her cancer was diagnosed, she was a senior writer at *People* magazine and finishing her book *Liaison: The Real Story of the Affair that Inspired 'M Butterfly'*.

My
Breast

ONE WOMAN'S CANCER STORY

JOYCE WADLER

Afterword by Susan M Love, MD

Published in Great Britain by The Women's Press Ltd, 1994
A member of the Namara Group
34 Great Sutton Street, London EC1V 0DX

First published in the United States of America by
Addison-Wesley Publishing Company, 1992

Reprinted 1994

Portions of this book have previously appeared in somewhat
different form in *New York* magazine. Some of the names in
this book have been changed to protect the privacy of those
involved.

British Library Cataloguing-in-Publication Data
A catalogue record for this book is available from
the British Library

ISBN 0 7043 4391 6

Typeset in 11½ point Berkeley Old Style

Printed and bound in Great Britain by
BPC Paperbacks Ltd, Aylesbury, Bucks

For Herb, for being there

My
Breast

I

I HAVE A SCAR ON MY LEFT BREAST, FOUR INCHES LONG, which runs from the right side of my breast to just above the nipple. Nick, who I no longer see, once said if anyone asked, I should say I was attacked by a jealous woman. The true story, which I prefer, is that a surgeon made the cut, following a line I had drawn for him the night before. He had asked me where I wanted the scar, and I had put on a black strapless bra and my favorite party dress and drawn a line in ink just below the top of the bra, a good four inches below the tumor. The surgeon took it out using a local, and when he was done, I asked to see it. It was the size of a robin's egg, with the gray brain-like matter which gives it its name, medullary cancer. It rested in the middle of a larger ball of pink and white breast tissue, sliced down the center like a hard-boiled egg, an onion-like layering of whitish-gray tissue about it, and I looked at it hard, trying to figure it out. We did not know it was cancer until twenty minutes later, when they had almost finished stitching me up and the pathology report came back, and then I was especially glad I had looked. *Mano a mano*, eyeball to eyeball. This is a modern story. Me and my cancer. I won.

I I

WHO DO I INTRODUCE FIRST, ME OR MY BREASTS? FORMERLY,
I thought of my body as a unit, indivisible, with my
breasts in some small way contributing to my notion of
who I am. Now, having shown the ability to destroy me, I
regard them with new respect, thinking perhaps they de-
serve not only separate but higher billing. As this is a
breast-cancer story, maybe they should have it.

They are, anyway, good-sized breasts, and though
they are fibrocystic, which means the milk-producing tissues tend to thicken and form fluid-filled sacs, and
though I have what some people claim may be other pre-
disposing factors for cancer—menstruation at an early
age, no children—I did not worry about the disease.
There is no history of breast cancer in my family; I do not
smoke; I go to the gym. My father, the year before my diagnosis, had died of prostate cancer, but I viewed this as a
separate thing. Also, because I knew it would be difficult
for me to spot a malignant lump, given the cystic condition of my breasts, I made sure my gynecologist always
examined them, and I had regular mammograms. I had

my first, at my doctor's suggestion, when I was thirty. For the last five years I had gone to the Guttman Breast Diagnostic Institute in Manhattan, which had been recommended to me by my gynecologist as being as good as a private service and a whole lot cheaper. In 1986 it was forty-five dollars, as opposed to ninety dollars; if a woman couldn't afford to pay, it was free. The wait was long, but there was a cozy female camaraderie, sitting in your paper hospital shirt next to ladies of all ages and seeing how many shapes we come in. One morning, when the room was exceptionally crowded, I counted up and figured out there were 140 breasts ahead of me. I had a mammogram once a year, and every year the letter I got afterward began the same:

"Dear Ms. Wadler,
    We are pleased to inform you that the results of your examination were satisfactory and within normal limits. . . ."

Who I am is a journalist, forty-four, Jewish, never married, which, as everybody in the United States knows, thanks to our eight billion collective hours of analysis, is a whole other category than single. I grew up in a large, noisy, opinionated family, in a boarding house in the

Catskills, a resort area which in the fifties was a good thirty years past its prime. The landscape was dotted with grand hotels with sagging porches and peeling paint; the population, during the summer, in what we called "the season," was largely New York City Jews, many of whom had concentration camp numbers tattooed on their arms. They bundled their children in jackets on the hottest days, dressed for dinner as they had in Vienna before the war, and spent their evenings at whichever hotel had the band, the women being particularly fond of Xavier Cugat and mink-trimmed sweaters and cha-cha. The lesson of the tattoos was not difficult to understand. My two younger brothers and I would have figured it out even if my mother hadn't repeated it to us, in perfect Wadler non sequitur three times a week: "You're lucky to be in America, because if you'd been born in Europe, you wouldn't have been born." The lure of Latin music would take me much longer to understand, though as a ten-year-old I wondered about it often: What on earth was it with Jews and cha-cha? It wasn't until my midthirties, when I started losing people myself, that I figured it out: The longer death casts a shadow, the faster you need to dance.

Our place, The Maplewood House, could not even claim to having once been a grand hotel. It was a dairy farm, expanded to boarding house with pool, and run by my father's mother, Gussie, who, rather than leaving the Russian province of Molov Guburney in 1913, brought it to America with her. It enclosed her like a capsule, the Bubbie in the Bubble; she never learned to read English and preferred to speak to me in Yiddish, a language I did not entirely understand. Her nickname among her in-laws in New York City was "the greena cousina," the greenhorn, because she was so innocent of the twentieth century that the first time she put her foot on the treadle of an electric sewing machine in a Lower East Side sweat-shop and encountered a machine that could move without being turned by hand, she fell to the floor in shock. Relocated to the mountains with her three sons and wid-owed, however, she ran the show. I remember her as a warm and powerful presence, dotted with flour: five feet six inches, 175 pounds; cooking for 120 people in a layer of cardigans and a man's white apron; or standing in the back of the kitchen, clanging an enormous iron bell and hollering to the help, "Boys, come eat." When she heard there was a new teacher in the neighboring town of Fleischmanns, and she was that rarest of off-season com-modities, a Jewish girl, she ordered her youngest son to go to a dance at the school and he did, ultimately marry-ing the girl. If she caught wind of a domestic dispute—for when I was small, we all lived in the same big house—she flung herself into the middle of it, thrusting her enormous chest forward, tearing open the uppermost of her two sweaters and screaming, "You wanna hit? You wanna hit? You wanna hit? If you want to hit, hit *me,* don't hit the children." It always stopped the action, because it was so preposterous. In my family, nobody ever hit. The aggression, such as it was, came all from the mouth. As for the family business, it was clear it was a style of life on the way out. Every fall, with the guests safely returned to the city and the insurance premiums paid, another hotel would go up in flames. My father, who was chief of the volunteer fire department, was not unsympathetic. "Save the trees!" he yelled, when the fire trucks arrived too fast.

I made my escape to New York, to Greenwich Village, at seventeen and have lived here ever since, working for newspapers and magazines: My first newspaper job, at twenty-four, was at the *New York Post,* a liberal, afternoon paper which in those days was the Columbo of New York City journalism—scruffy and amiable, happy to sit on the stoop and schmooze. It was located on the East River, near the Brooklyn Bridge, with a grubby city room and an atmosphere a lot like the boarding house: noisy, histrionic, completely lacking in privacy, restraint, and tact. Staff was divided into two categories—Schreibers, who were the feature writers and tended to be moody and get stomach aches on deadline, and Reporters, who could dictate a hard news story from a phone booth with five minutes to go and strut off like a marine.

I was a Schreiber, writing stories about movie stars, kids raising pigeons on the roof, and convicts wrongly accused. At a paper which continued to do stories claiming Julius and Ethel Rosenberg had been railroaded twenty years after their execution for passing hydrogen-bomb secrets to the Soviets, convicts, unless they were landlords, were usually wrongly accused. The toughest thing the *Post* made me do was review the Yiddish theater, though by then I remembered maybe forty words. The show was *Shver Tsu Zayn a Yid* (*It's Hard to Be a Jew*) by Sholem Aleichem.

"They don't even have a translation; what am I supposed to do?" I asked the city editor.

"Rave," he said.

Herb, my closest friend, who today is a comedy writer, was a Schreiber, too. I looked up one day, and there he was across the city room—a tall, thin Jewish guy with a beard and a nice, slow smile. "All I know is his name is Levine, he comes from the *Baltimore Sun,* and they say he can make tapioca fascinating," I heard one of the other Schreibers say. Schreibers were a competitive bunch; a dazzling lead on somebody else's story could throw your ordinary Schreiber into a funk for the afternoon, but somehow nobody was jealous of Herb. His stuff was so tight, so funny, it was simply accepted that he was in another league. He had a neat, off-angle way of coming at a story, too. When they sent him to do a feature about a trapeze artist who was doing her act suspended from a crane in midtown Manhattan, he ignored the girl and interviewed the crane operator. When they made him interview a hundred-and-three-year-old lady and ask her the secret of her long life—a tabloid staple—he wrote the story without mentioning her age. He was a quiet guy. In a newspaper cafeteria with great storytellers elbowing for center stage, he might throw in one sentence; but when he talked, he was the funniest man in New York. For a while, in my twenties, we went out, but it soon became clear that much as he liked women, Herb liked solitude more. He also saw no need to perpetuate the race, which he viewed much as my family viewed the boarding house: a low-rent undertaking which was doomed.

"We could get married," I said to him one day. "We could have babies. I would raise them."

"And I would lower them," said Herb.

After that, we went back to friends. Now we hang out so much that when I am seeing somebody, we joke about how to explain about Herb. Herb's idea is to throw a sheet over him when he is lying on the couch reading the papers, and after each date I pull back the sheet a little bit, and by the time it gets serious, the guy understands about Herb.

At the time this story begins, I had had a lot of serious dates and a lot of jobs and was working as a writer at *People* magazine. If, as research claims, tension contributes to disease, I was a good candidate: I had been working, for the last two years, on a book on a French espionage case, juggling six-month stays in Paris with a staff job in New York. Though the case, which had inspired the Broadway show *M. Butterfly*, was wonderful, Paris when I first arrived had been hard. There is a mythology involving Paris one does not encounter if doing a book in Cleveland. It is expected, even from people who have been around, that you will have a great love affair and red geraniums in a window box, and Gene Kelly will come whistling down the *quai*. In fact, though I bought the geraniums the day after my arrival and walked along the Seine looking for Gene, moving to Paris was relocating alone to a strange town. I had two friends. I did not speak French. I sometimes went entire Sundays speaking only to waiters. Soon after I returned from my first stay in France, my father died a prolonged and ugly death, hooked up to a life-support machine. I was a bad fit at

People and always had been: I like forty inches just to say hello. The style at *People,* which I had come to respect as one does a skill which does not come easily, was somewhere between sausage and haiku: reduce *War and Peace* to a snappy two pager, and then if Photo can't get a home-take of Pierre and Natasha in the hot tub, they kill the story anyway. I could do it, but it made my head hurt. I was tired all the time. On weekends and evenings I wrote my book; during the day I went to the magazine.

Also, I was in a difficult relationship. His name was Nick Di Stefano. He was a newspaper guy I had known for years, and I had been seeing him, on and off, for eight months, since the summer. He was Italian, which in my family is considered practically Jewish, except that (1) as children, Italians don't talk back to their parents, and (2) as adults, the men Run Around. Naturally, being so troublesome, we find them very appealing, and anyway, I had always liked Nick. He was smart; he knew all the lyrics to *The Pajama Game*; he dressed like a forties sharpie; he had the requisite newspaper up-yours attitude regarding authority. Also, there is something very nice about a relationship where you have known each other a long time and are in the same business. We watched old movies from his collection, and he cooked and told me what an exceptional woman his mother was and took me dancing. Then he waltzed off to Miami for a weekend with an old girlfriend, and that was the end of Nick, The First Chapter. She, it turned out, wanted to be just friends. Now when Nick is with me, he is often petulant, seeing himself as the tragic hero of a doomed love affair, a role I have traditionally tried to reserve for myself.

"Why does it always have to be so serious with you?" he says. "Why can't we just live in the moment?"

And also, "You don't want me to work it out and decide what's right for me. You just think if you give me enough time I'll get her out of my system."

"That's what you want in a woman, to be that selfless—you should be dating Mother Teresa," I say. "Why don't you call her up in Calcutta and see if she's available. From what you tell me, she's the only single woman you haven't nailed."

Then we break up and I go to bed depressed and lose two days out of my book.

That's where we're at, broken up, the morning I discover the lump. It is the first week in March, a Monday, one of the craziest days of the week at *People*. I am feeling particularly tense because I'm taking another leave of absence and have one week in which to finish my outstanding stories. I am so frantic, I have canceled my mammogram at the Guttman the week before, figuring I'll do it when my leave begins.

Then, as I'm showering, I feel it: a large, egg-shaped swelling on the upper, inner part of my left breast. I have always wondered how women who discover lumps find them, but there is no missing this: it seems to be, as I move my hand around it, the size of an egg, slightly raised, sore to the touch. My breasts, since my midthirties, have been sore and swollen before my period, and as I've gotten older the soreness has increased—a normal part of aging, which will increase until menopause, a doctor has told me—but I had my period two weeks ago. Another strange thing: this lump seems so big, and I don't remember it being there yesterday. I decide I should probably get it checked out, but I am not very concerned. What I have heard about breast cancer is that except for finding a lump, it is asymptomatic—you don't have pain. I figure it's just another one of my fibrocystic lumps, which come and go. I'll call the Guttman and be sure to make that appointment for next week.

I go to work and forget about it. Then in the afternoon my breast starts to ache. I remember that *People* has a staff doctor and call him up. I feel a little silly about this; I am sure it is nothing, but I figure a doctor is right there in the building, so why not? He doesn't seem worried either, until he examines me. Then his face seems to tighten up. In the bright light of the examining room, where there is a small mirror, I think I see why: there is a pink flush on my breast in the area of the lump, which I did not see at home, as if there is an inflammation. There is definitely something there, the doctor says. What it is, he cannot say, but he thinks I should see a specialist. If I like, he'll be glad "to expedite it." I tell him I'm planning to have my regular mammogram at the Guttman next week.

"I think it would be better if you saw somebody sooner than that," he says. He repeats himself. "If I can, I would like to set something up for you."

I burst into tears.

Boy, I think, I really must be strung tight today. And to him, though he hasn't mentioned the word that is now as much a presence in the room as another human being, "Sorry. My father died of cancer last year."

He makes a call. An hour later, I am standing outside the Time-Life Building, hailing a cab for the Upper East Side offices of a surgeon we'll call Luke. I am scared. Before I left his office, the doctor asked me if I would have health coverage during my leave, and that has added to my feeling that this is serious. I am now flip-flopping between telling myself that I am overreacting and a kind of giddy hysteria. Standing on Sixth Avenue, I have turned into Zorba the Greek. I want to *live*. The things I haven't done flash before me, a long list of "But wait, I wanna . . .": But wait, I wanna finish my book; but wait, I wanna get married; but wait, I wanna make some money and take Nick to Paris to meet my friends; but wait, I'm just getting started. . . . I think about Nick and the time we've wasted fighting and make a deal with myself: If everything's okay, I won't worry about monogamy; I won't *hock* him about moving in. I will make the most of every moment. Unwittingly as Newton discovered gravity, I have stumbled upon the key to making me the dream girl of every uncommitted man in Manhattan: breast cancer.

In the doctor's office there are at least a dozen women. They seem somewhat older than me, and oddly, they all look alike. They look like a truck ran over their faces, I find myself thinking, which I know, as soon as it crosses my mind, is an ugly thought and not correct. Then I realize what I am looking at: fear. I have never seen so much of it sitting together. It's a good thing there's nothing wrong with *me,* I think. Then, as I have a long wait, I go out for a walk. I have already called Herb, but now I find I want to talk to Nick, too. He tells me that it is probably nothing and not to get upset, and he is very sweet.

"Just tell me what you want me to do, baby," he says.

The doctor, when I get in to see him, is my age, blond and WASPy, a good listener, with the kind of calm I like to see in airline pilots and other people to whom I am entrusting my life. Speaking to him, I remember something: In the past few months, in addition to soreness before my period, my breasts have been sore afterward. They were so sensitive that it was uncomfortable for me if Nick rested his head on my chest—now that I think about it, the left side of my chest—and I wondered if I had had a false period and was pregnant. Nick and I sometimes played a little fast and loose with birth control, and though it wasn't supposed to be on the agenda, I would have liked very much for us to have a baby. Though I had called my gynecologist's office and asked a nurse if it really was possible to be pregnant, yet have a period, it never occurred to me to make an appointment and have the doctor check my breasts—she had examined them four months before.

Now, Luke examines me.

"I don't think this is anything to worry about," he says, and I feel relief rushing over me like a warm bath. "Malignancies tend to be hard, almost stony. You can't manipulate them. This you can. I'm 98 percent sure this is not malignant."

16

What he believes I have, Luke says, is an inflammation of some sort, perhaps an infected cyst. To find out, he would like to aspirate the lump—stick in a hypodermic, take out some liquid, and send it off to a lab to be analyzed—painless; all I'll feel is a needle prick. When a cyst is aspirated, a lot of liquid usually comes out. It *is* painless, but it doesn't go as planned.

"Huh, that's odd," he says, and he shows me: He has been able to draw out very little liquid, which should not be the case if it's a cyst. What liquid there is, however, is thick and puslike, which is consistent with infection.

I get dressed and we talk. Luke tells me he still sees no reason for concern at this time. I do: "If it's a cyst," I ask, "how come more liquid didn't come out? And if it's not a cyst, what is it?"

"I don't know," says Luke. "That's why we're doing the tests."

I go meet Nick at The Lion's Head, a writers' hangout in the Village. He's wearing his fedora low on his head and gives me that cocky Bronx grin that has always knocked me out.

"See, I knew it would be nothing," he says, and within hours we are un-broken up.

III

I AM NOT A HYPOCHONDRIAC. I LEAN TOWARD THE OTHER EX-
treme, a person who associates sickness with weakness
and therefore denies being sick. This, I believe, is the le-
gacy of my mother, Milly, who ran off to Florida at seventeen to paint flamingos on glass; in my childhood stole
trees from state forest preserves, insisting they were hers
because her tax dollars had paid for them; and at sixty-
five is still one of the great forces of nature on the East
Coast.

"I've never been sick a day in my life," she says. "One
hour after I had you, I was eating. The other women in
the hospital were screaming their heads off. I took one
look at them and made up my mind, 'How it went in, it
will go out,' and that was that. This worrying you have
about every little thing, that you got from your father. He
was the worrier. Him and his mother. The Aspirin Ad-
dict."

Also, before going off at sixty-two to serve as a volunteer in the Israeli army:

"I don't fear death. Death to me is just another adventure. I can think of no greater honor than dying for the state of Israel, the Jewish homeland."

"You're an old dame, Ma," I say. "Whadaya think— they're gonna put a machine gun in your hand and send you to the front? You're gonna be cleaning toilets."

"Don't even bother to bring back the body," she says.

I do fear death. Even more, now, I fear a bad death, strapped up to machines in a hospital, like my father. "Joyce," he had taken to telling me from the mountains, when I called once a week from Paris, "your father is a very sick man. Your father is dying." I did not entirely believe him. I knew he was sick, very sick. I had been there for the early operations in the city and the last-minute flights to Florida. I knew the cancer was creeping up his spine and down his legs and was eventually going to kill him. But his blood counts were good, he was going to his business every day. It is a rotten thing to admit, but a voice in me, hearing him, was satirizing him: "Joyce, Your Father is dying"—Hebraic Dramatic Third Person, now replacing that previous family favorite, "You realize, of course, you are killing your father."

He was a worrier, too, and critical and angry: worrying how he and his mother and his two younger brothers would survive in a run-down boarding house when he was seventeen and his father died; worrying about making a new business out of nothing when he was in his thirties and boarding houses were going out; worrying once he was successful it would all disappear. Then, when I got home from Paris, I saw the worrying was real: my father was sixty-seven and got up from his desk at the office like a man of eighty-five, his weight down thirty pounds, shaking, supporting himself on a cane. Seeing me, he started to cry. "I never thought I'd see you again," he said, and I was filled with self-loathing. "What the fuck was I doing in Paris all that time? I didn't even need all of that stuff. Why wasn't I here with my father?" Two weeks later he took a fall and broke his hip, and after that operation his heart started to fail, and they put him on life support. "You're not getting enough oxygen, Bernie," the doctor said. "Your lungs are exhausting your heart. If we don't put you on this machine, you're going to die. Do you give your consent?" and my father nodded yes. Nobody in the family had any idea what life support meant, but in an hour, when they let us in to see him, we found out. An oxygen tube had been stuffed down his nose and was taped across his face; his hands were strapped to the side of the hospital bed; he was pulling against the straps like an animal at auction, trying to speak but unable to because of the tube down his throat.

"We had to tie his hands to the bed because he already pulled the tube out of his nose once already," one of the doctors said. "He's a little out of it now because we sedated him."

He was on the machine for two months. A few days into it they gave him a tracheotomy so he would be more comfortable, but he could never again speak. I knew it was his life and going on the machines had been his decision, but I never changed my mind about it. I think he would have been better off dead.

I do not, however, dwell on that memory the week of the scare. I trust Dr. Luke and I know he's good—a journalist friend was a patient and says his reputation is excellent; he's known among doctors who treat Presidents. I do mention the lump to my mother, who is in Florida for the winter, but I tell her I don't think it's anything serious, and I believe it.

That changes a little on Thursday when I talk to Luke about the test results. He tells me, in a tone indicating there is nothing to be concerned about, that what they see is mostly material that looks like inflammation and not cancer, "though they do see some breast cells that look atypical."

My old reporter's bell goes off.

"What do you mean 'atypical'?" I ask. "How many cells?"

He seems a bit irritated by the question, as if I'm worrying for no reason.

"Atypical does not mean cancer," he says. "But it does not mean normal either. This can happen with an inflammation."

He prescribes Dicloxacillin, 500 milligrams, four tablets daily, to see if that reduces the swelling. He also says that he thinks the best thing to do is a biopsy and take the lump out—but first, let's see how it responds to the drugs.

The next week, I start my leave. Though *People* and I have our problems, in this area they have been extraordinarily good to me. This is my third leave in three years; it includes medical benefits. I am perhaps eighty pages away from finishing my book, and it is a story about which a writer dreams: A young French foreign service worker, posted to China on the eve of the Cultural Revolution, falls in love with a strange and secretive Chinese opera singer and becomes a spy for the Chinese to protect her life. They have a son. Eighteen years later, after finally getting his mistress and child to France, the singer and spy are arrested and charged with espionage. In prison the Frenchman, whose name is Bernard Boursicot, is suddenly confronted with the news that the woman he loves is a man. Nobody believes he could not have known. His own mother seems to have doubts. "He was drunk, right?" she asked me, the first time we were alone; but I've spent three years with Bernard, and I know what the real story is.

I have also come to like Bernard very much. He is not the sexually repressed *fonctionnaire* I feared he might be when I first got interested in the story. He's a wild man who views the world as a smorgasbord at which it is impossible to overeat. He is also even more of a movie-mad romantic than Nick—which is, in part, what got him into all that trouble in the first place. He's seen *Dr. Zhivago* thirteen times, being particularly susceptible to wide-screen dramas. He relishes having been a spy, making toasts to Philby, Burgess, and Meredith whenever he encounters a Brit he wants to tweak. He excels at cinematic gesture. "I shall pick you up at the airport playing 'April in Paris,'" he told me, the spring I was scheduled to first arrive. Sure enough, after we'd piled my luggage into his little Citroën at Orly, he hit the tape deck and there came Ella Fitzgerald, promising chestnuts in blossom, and my broad-shouldered spy in his trench coat looked over at me and grinned. Journalistically, he could be quite draining. "God has cursed me with the one person in the universe more operatic than myself," I wrote Herb after one five-hour interview, for Bernard had taken some heavy losses, and his melancholy moods were black. When he turned on the charm, however, nobody could resist. "You know, I saw the play *M. Butterfly* in New York when it first opened, and when the opera singer turned out to be a man, I was amazed," a visiting girlfriend told him one night over dinner. "Me, too," said Bernard, pouring her some more wine and sizing her up the way the other people in the restaurant were eyeing dessert. Writing his story has been the most difficult and satisfying assignment of my life, and it's getting better all the time. My twenty-four-year-old assistant, Stephane, back in Paris, has cornered a source we've wanted for two years. I'm coming up on the most terrifying and dramatic moments in Bernard's life, when he will confront his lover about the deception and later attempt suicide.

The only thing is, I am so distracted by this thing in my chest, I am having trouble concentrating on my book. It's so sore I cannot sleep on my stomach. The penicillin, which at first seemed to be reducing both the pain and the lump, doesn't seem to be doing much after ten days. There is a very bright light in my gym locker room, and I see how vivid and delineated the area around the lump still is.

"I'm starting to feel this thing has a life of its own," I tell Herb one night, as he's stretched out on the couch.

"Like it's gonna come flying out of my body any minute, like that thing in *Alien*, and run around the living room and put on the sports channel and ask for a beer."

I decide it's time for independent research and pull out my two medical reference books. My old stand-by, *The A.M.A. Family Medical Guide*, is not very comforting: It defines *breast abscess* as a pus-filled infected area but says that it is uncommon and usually affects women who are breast-feeding. It says, starting to make me nervous, that a cancerous lump "may or may not be painful," that it occurs most often in women in their forties and fifties and is "slightly more common in women who have never breast-fed a baby." The only good news I can see is that it is also "slightly more common" in women whose families have a history of the disease. The *Professional Guide to Diseases*, a handy reporter's tool, is even worse. It adds white, middle- and upper-class women to their higher-risk list, as well as those "who are under constant stress and undergo unusual disturbances in their home and work lives."

Eleven days after the discovery of the lump, I go back to see Dr. Luke. He examines my breast and in less than a minute makes a decision.

"This has to come out," he says.

I am not scared now; I am relieved. I don't think it's

cancer—I'm too healthy for cancer—I just want this thing out of my body, the sooner the better. I'd be happy if he could do it right now in the office. He says that's out of the question. It will be done with a local anesthetic at a hospital and will take maybe half an hour, forty-five minutes. I ask if I will be able to watch: I saw breast surgery when I did a story on a plastic surgeon in Beverly Hills, and I also hung out for a month at the New York City morgue, so I figure I won't be squeamish. Luke says he'll be glad to explain as he cuts, but that most people do not want to watch when theirs is the body involved. I decide he's right.

I also realize I am concerned about a scar. I've never considered myself particularly vain; I had always thought of scars as a badge of honor, a sign of a battle vanquished, but those, I now realize, were scars on other people. Luke says he can get to the lump from any number of spots—just show him where to make the cut. He books the surgery for five days later. I have one last problem.

"I've got this deadline on this book," I say. "This isn't going to hang me up time-wise, is it?"

"Listen," he says, "this comes first. This is your life."

A few friends, in addition to my brothers and my shrink, by now know I have a lump in my breast and am starting to worry about it, but it is Herb I ask to come to the hospital. He is a free-lance, while Nick works nine to five. More importantly, after the initial enthusiasm which accompanies all our reconciliations, Nick, as usual, is preoccupied with his own problems—an apartment he cannot unload in a depressed real estate market, his unrequited passion. He loves me, he has said shortly before our last breakup; we do get along wonderfully, particularly in the sack, but what we have is really a friendship. His old girlfriend, he says forlornly, is his "sickness," his "obsession." It's madness, he tells me; I am better than her in every way; it makes sense that we are together, but feelings are feelings. "'What fools these mortals be,'" he has taken to saying. "'What fools.' Mickey Rooney as Puck, *Midsummer Night's Dream*. You've never seen it? You're kidding. His intonation was perfect—the way he said it: 'What *fools*.'" Given this, I am reluctant to ask Nick for anything. Also, Nick hates doctors. Who goes to doctors?, says Nick. Women. Something is wrong—the best thing you can do is leave it alone, and it will fix itself. In my case, we don't even know that anything is wrong, so let's just quit thinking about it. I think I know the real reason: Nick's first wife, the mother of his twenty-four-year-old son, who developed schizophrenia in her early thirties. She had been a nurse, the head of a department; when she realized, in one of her increasingly rare moments of lucidity, what was happening to her mind, she killed herself. It follows, Nick cannot deal with loss. I give up trying to talk about my breast with Nick and take a stroll by myself to Barnes & Noble, to the section where they have the medical textbooks. The most comprehensive seems to be *Breast Cancer, Conservative and Reconstructive Surgery* by Bohmert, Leis, and Jackson, a collection of studies. It's $129, too much to spend if I don't even know I have a problem, but I skim it, looking at the pictures. There are a lot of women squooshing a breast like they are squeezing the Charmin. I figure it's to show how lifelike reconstructions have become, but it strikes me as a man's notion of what is important to a woman. I have never in my life squooshed my breast that hard, and if a man did it, I would holler. I flip through the studies. Every one seems to include a figure about five-year survival rates. I put the book away.

The night before surgery I spend alone. Nick calls three times, asking when I am leaving for the hospital so he can call and wish me well. I remember I have to make my decision about the scar. I put on a bandeau bra that is the skimpiest I own and a skinny little Nicole Miller dress, deep purple, with spaghetti straps, that I wore one night when Nick took me to the Rainbow Room, soon after we'd started dating. I loved that night. I had a thirties evening bag that I had gotten for forty francs at a flea market in Paris, a deco rhinestone bracelet from an estate sale in New York, and as I got dressed, I wondered about the women who had owned the bag and the bracelet and where they had worn them and if they had been as happy as me. Then I take off the dress and turn down the top of the bra and trace the edge with a ballpoint pen. As I do, I start to cry. I don't have a perfect body by model standards; my breasts are different from what they were in my twenties; I did, when I watched the plastic surgeon, have a fantasy of a lift. But they are my breasts; it is my body— I like it very much. Now I am making a mark that says, Cut me.

Early the next morning, I talk to Nick. "Call me with the good news as soon as you get out of surgery," he says. Then Herb and I head up to Roosevelt, a private, voluntary hospital in a rough, working-class neighborhood in Manhattan that used to be called Hell's Kitchen. I've chosen Roosevelt because Luke has told me there is little paperwork for outpatient procedures and I can get in and out fast, but I'm not crazy about it. I spent an evening there years ago, doing a story on a New York City Emergency Medical Ambulance team, and I remember it as a run-down, depressing place with an overcrowded waiting room and derelicts at the door. I also once visited a friend in her late fifties who had just had a malignant lump removed from her breast and was a patient at the hospital. She had known about the lump for six months, a friend told me, and would not see a doctor. We were not close, but there were two things about the visit that struck me: She would not admit to us she had known about the lump and ignored it. Instead she talked for twenty minutes, in what seemed to be pointless and obsessive detail, about what she claimed to have thought was a tennis injury, a pulled muscle in her chest—bothersome, but not enough to see a doctor. Why is she telling us this? I thought as the story dragged on, until it dawned on me: she was trying to justify to herself her delay in getting medical help. I also remember that she had been given as a roommate a woman who was dying of breast cancer. The woman drifted in and out of consciousness, moaning, and I wondered how anyone could have made such an insensitive match. Within two years, my friend was dead too.

Now, in the taxi, in the ten-minute ride to Roosevelt, I push that memory aside and recall all the strange trips I have taken with Herb: Kenya, where we eyed the lions from an open Land Rover and got scared they were seeing two New York Jews and getting an urge for delicatessen; Paris, where we went looking for Jim Morrison's grave at

Père-Lachaise Cemetery and had no idea where to find it until we spotted a girl with a ring in her nose and pink hair. Now I tell Herb we should regard this as just another weird adventure.

"You sure you don't want to come in and watch the surgery—not that I know that they'd let you—because it could be kind of interesting," I say.

"Pass," says Herb.

Roosevelt, on Ninth Avenue, is as gloomy as I remember. A group of homeless people have set up housekeeping to one side of the building, on West Fifty-eighth Street, arranging a sofa and two armchairs in traditional living-room style. Inside, it looks like it hasn't been painted for years. On the third-floor short-term-stay center, Herb parks himself in a reception area while I go to a large room, which is partitioned with curtains, and change into baggy hospital clothes. Taking off my bra, I see that the line I have drawn is very low, nearly halfway down my breast. "Wonderful," I think. "Now the doctor is going to think I'm fast." A few minutes later, the surgical resident who will be assisting Luke drops by.

"Whoa! You can't miss that!" he says when he touches the lump.

A few minutes later an orderly takes me to the surgery waiting room, and Luke comes to get me. He looks very preppie, sockless in clogs, and is very sweet, putting an arm around my shoulder as we walk to the operating room. I have a feeling this is politically incorrect behavior and I am not supposed to like it, but I do. The operating team includes two nurses, a man and a woman, as well as the resident and Luke. Seeing the line on my breast, Luke laughs.

"You've sure made this idiot-proof," he says.

They paint my left breast with a red ointment that smells like iodine and cover the rest of my chest with sterile cloth. I can't see the surgery itself, because Luke has asked me to turn my face to the right; but as he has promised, he tells me what I will feel and what he is doing as he moves along. The painkiller is Xylocaine. He injects it at various points around my breast, waiting for the area to numb; then he makes a cut. I have a feeling of warmth and wetness. Then there are strong sensations of tugging, as he pulls back tissue and starts tunneling up from the incision to the lump, in the inner upper quadrant of my breast. Sometimes I feel a bit of pain, almost a burning sensation, and he gives me more Xylocaine. The tunneling seems to go on for twenty minutes, and while it is not as uncomfortable as a dentist's drilling, the more tissue that is being pulled apart and clamped, the more uncomfortable I become. I am having second thoughts now about being so concerned about looking good in a low-cut dress. Luke tells me they've reached the lump, but they're going to go a little beyond it, to make sure they've got it all by getting a good margin of healthy tissue from all sides. I'm starting, now, to get worried again. I don't know whether the room is cool or I'm feeling a nervous chill, but Luke seems to be cutting a lot of flesh—I know the lump is high, but I feel he is burrowing up toward my collarbone. Then I feel some final tugging and the thing is out, and I see out of the corner of my eye a metal tray, and then they are cauterizing blood vessels. Luke moves away from the operating table and a few minutes later comes back. It's a tumor all right, he says, his voice sounding serious, but what sort he cannot say. He's sending it down to the lab now. I tell him before he does, I'd like to see.

"You sure?" he says.

"Yeah," I say.

I turn my head and he picks it up. I am astonished at how big it is, how much tissue has been taken out of my breast. The excised flesh is the size of a tangerine and has been sliced cleanly down the middle through the tumor—that must be what Luke was doing when he briefly left the table. The inside, which is the size of a robin's egg, is grayish-white, covered with a layer of whitish-pink tissue. Around that is what appears to me to be normal breast tissue, pink and white, like very fatty, coarsely ground chopped meat. Luke points out the layering around the tumor, telling me it appears to be encapsulated, and that is good. I don't think any of this is good. I can't believe this big gray glob came out of me; I have a very bad feeling, a sense of unreality, as if I am in a dream or a place I have no desire to be.

"How soon will we know the results?" I say, as they start stitching me up.

"About twenty minutes," Luke says.

And then, more to myself than to anyone else: "How am I going to tell my mother?"

"Don't get yourself worked up," the male nurse says. "We don't even know that it's anything yet," and I try to hold on to that thought. But another part of me thinks he's patronizing me; maybe they don't want to deal with the possibility of a flipped-out woman on the table if they've got to stitch up her chest. I feel lonely, unable to talk about what I'm thinking about, and scared. I try to concentrate on being calm. In what seems to be fifteen minutes, just as they've finished cleaning me up and bandaging me, somebody comes into the room.

"Well, it is a tumor and it *is* malignant," Luke begins briskly, as if he's giving a lecture to a group of medical students. "It's what's called a medullary carcinoma. It's . . ."

I am having trouble following. Thoughts are going through my head faster than I was aware thoughts could travel: This can't be real. Is he telling me I'm going to die? Should I ask for a rabbi? No, wait, I'm not a religious Jew, I'm more like an ethnic Jew, that would be hypocritical, but maybe rabbis in hospitals are more like therapists. Why is he telling me this stuff here, where I'm alone? Wasn't that the point of bringing Herb?

I interrupt him.

"Do you think we could hold off on this until we get upstairs and you can talk to my friend, too?" I say.

And, as we head to the third-floor waiting room, "I think I could use a drink."

They offer me a wheelchair, but I don't want it—it is very important for me to be on my feet. Herb is where I left him. I have slowly been formulating the idea that it will be bad to be negative, that I'm under attack and it's got to be all systems go; but as I see Herb, I give him a thumbs down and shake my head. Luke takes us into one of the little curtained-off cubicles.

"It's, like, malignant," I say.

Herb looks dazed. We find chairs. A nurse, hearing

what is going on, silently brings me a cup of coffee, a small gesture that is enormously comforting. Luke starts his talk from the top. I had remembered from my father's illness that it is important to take notes when you see the doctor, because in times of stress you do not remember all you hear. My notebook is in a locker with my clothes, but I see Herb, stunned as he is, pull his little notebook out of his blazer and start writing, as if it's the old days and he's at a press conference. I feel a wave of love. He's so solid. I focus in on Luke. He is saying that they've removed a medullary cancer, which is a relatively infrequent type, with "a better-than-average prognosis." It was "a well-circumscribed mass," 2.8 centimeters, with seemingly clean tissue around it—he'll have more detailed results in a few days. It has been caught early: clinically, it's a stage-two cancer. Provided there is no cancer in the lymph nodes under the arm, it is really "quite curable." I do not entirely believe him. I was in the room with my father when a New York specialist told him that prostate cancer was curable. Four years later, he was dead. On the other hand, this is all so weird, I don't know what to believe. I don't even know if what I say next is me or something I picked up from the movies. I just feel it's important to get it straight.

"Look," I say, "I have no plans of dying of this thing. That's just not how I see my life. So what's the next step?"

Luke runs through them: The next thing to do is remove some lymph nodes from under my left arm and see if the cancer has spread. That's very important—the key diagnostic tool. We also have to decide how we want to treat the breast: with lumpectomy and radiation or with mastectomy and reconstruction. Lumpectomy is removing the tumor and leaving the breast, which is what he has just done, except that he would reopen the incision to take another look. The success rates for lumpectomy and mastectomy, he says, are the same. Either way you go, lumpectomy or mastectomy, the lymph nodes have to come out. I have another terror besides death—general anesthesia. I am afraid that even if I survive, my brain will not.

"This lymph-node surgery, can it be done under a local?" I ask him.

"Impossible," he says.

I remember lymph nodes. When they took a sampling from my father's groin, there was cancer in eight out of eleven. I didn't know what that meant then, but I knew it was bad: the surgeon, calling Dad's room after the operation, asked to speak to me, not to my mother.

"What are the chances it's in the lymph nodes?" I ask Luke.

"Twenty to 30 percent," he says.

I'm feeling a little dreamlike again. I don't get it, I tell Luke. I had mammograms; I had checkups. This thing was enormous—how was it missed? He tells me medullary is not like other cancers—it may not calcify and can appear on a mammogram as another cyst.

"So how do we know there's not another one of these things somewhere inside me?" I say.

"We don't," he says. "Your breasts are a breast surgeon's nightmare. They're large and dense and full of lumps."

I don't know what breast reconstruction involves, but I remember the pictures in the medical book. If the real ones are gonna be this dangerous, let them make me a fake.

"Take it off," I say.

He talks a little about breast reconstruction. I had figured it would be somewhat like the breast-augmentation surgery I had seen in L.A.: a one-step procedure where they knock you out, slip in an implant, and you wake up with a new breast—except that with cancer, they would take out the breast tissue first. Luke says it is not that simple: he would take out the breast tissue at the same time he removed the lymph nodes, but rebuilding the breast would take several months. You do that, you don't need to radiate the breast tissue—it's gone. Radiation treatment takes six weeks. Whether or not the cancer is in the nodes, there's a good chance I'll need chemotherapy drugs for six months.

I have never thought much about cancer, but one thing I have in my head is that if cancer is found in your body, you are supposed to move very quickly, perhaps within days. Luke tells me this is not the case, but that I should wait no longer than four weeks to have the lymph-node surgery. Meanwhile, they'll be doing more tests on the tumor: DNA analysis, estrogen receptors, something called a paraffin test. I can take the cotton dressing off my breast tomorrow; come to his office Friday, he'll have those results and take out the stitches. I'm having trouble assimilating all this, and from the look on his face, so is Herb. We're two liberal-arts guys suddenly thrown into Columbia Medical School. I'm still back with the news that breast reconstruction is a long-term process and I could be walking around lopsided for several months. Luke sees we're lost. Probably everybody, at this stage, is lost. He recommends a few books.

I have one more question. I am afraid to ask it, but it seems to want to come out of me anyway.

"What am I looking at here?" I ask. "Statistically?"

Luke doesn't seem to be any happier answering than I am asking. He doesn't care much for statistics, he says. You can still have a cancer that statistically has a high cure rate, and if you're in the percentage rate that is not cured, it doesn't matter. In my case, I have a cancer that has a favorable prognosis and is more curable than average.

I need something harder.

"When my father was diagnosed with prostate cancer, I checked the statistics, and it was something like a 60 percent survival rate at four years, a 40 percent survival rate at seven years," I say.

"I would say the statistics in your case are considerably better than that," Luke says.

"How much better?"

"For breast cancer, the overall cure rate is 70 percent in ten years; for medullary, it's well above that—I would say 80 percent, 90 percent."

I feel better. I like these odds. I'm not sure I believe them, but I like them. This leaves me with one immediate problem: how to tell my mother. Herb has the solution: Lead with the positive. I get dressed and find my notebook, and we work out the lead and phone it in. The last time I did this, it occurs to me, I was filing a breaking story for the *Washington Post* on a Concerto for Piano and

Dog at Carnegie Recital Hall. The dog had stage fright, which was good for me, as it gave me a new top. There is a reason people hate reporters. The phone rings and I begin the performance.

"Well, Ma, I'm out of surgery and I'm here at the hospital and everything went great," I say.

"Oh, thank God, I'm so relieved, I don't know what to say. I was so nervous I couldn't sit still, my friends called, I told everybody, 'Get off, get off, I can't talk, my daughter is right now this minute having surgery in New York. . . .'"

I break through the wall of words, power talking, a skill I developed from forty-three years of training with champions.

"The lump turned out to be malignant, but it's the best kind you can have," I say. "It's called medullary; it tends not to spread; they seem to have gotten it all. It was in one lump, I saw it, it looks like it was encapsulated—that's a good sign."

Silence. She believes me like I believe the doctors.

"I'm coming north," she says.

I tell her she is staying put, I probably won't be having surgery for at least a month, and hit her with all the other positive stuff I can think of. This cancer is very rare, hardly anybody gets it, and it has a very, very good prognosis. Yeah, it was big, but this kind grows very fast and, the doctor says, was caught early. The longer I talk, the harder it is. I am hearing my mother and my dead grandmothers and all the aunts in the family: "The worst thing in the world that can happen, the very worst thing, is for a parent to survive a child," they are saying.

"Talk to Herb, Ma," I say and walk down the hall.

Then I pull it together and call Nick. Most of our relationship, I've wanted him to be more expressive. Often, when we are together, he withdraws and watches two or three old movies in a row—if he doesn't, he says, he'll think about his life, which he can't bear. In the morning, he moves the television so that he can watch "Lucy" reruns from the shower. Right now, however, I have this feeling that if he falls apart, I will fall apart, and I need him to be strong.

"I'm going to tell you something, and I don't want you to get emotional, because it's going to sound worse than it probably is," I say.

I have the feeling, at the other end of the line, of a man who has been slugged in the stomach.

"You just got to give me a minute; I wasn't expecting this," he says.

Then Herb and I head downtown. Standing on

Ninth Avenue, I can't shake the feeling I have fallen into a dream.

"This seems really surreal to me," I tell him. "Take a cab to the hospital, they cut out a cancer, take a cab home. It has this sort of Drive-and-Deposit feel. Maybe it could be some kind of medical chain."

"You're taking this very well," Herb says.

"I don't know," I tell him. "When Luke told me it was malignant, I said I wanted a drink. Now he probably thinks I'm an alcoholic."

"It's a special occasion," says Herb. "I'm sure he understands."

Normally, a glass of wine puts me to sleep. Now, we go to The Lion's Head, to the back room, where we are known as The Ones Who Only Eat, and I order a margarita, then a second one. Then I talk tactics with Herb. The position I am taking, I say, is not that I have cancer, but that I *had* a cancer and they cut it out of me. I am not doing an avoidance number, we are going to research the hell out of this and get the best people in the business, but until it is established otherwise, I consider myself a healthy person. I go tottering off to my place. I am not sure now whether the sense of unreality is coming from the news I have received or the drinks. The Xylocaine is wearing off, and with every step, even in a bra and bandages, my breast bounces and hurts. Luke had offered me a prescription of Tylenol 3, but I'm a little afraid of drugs and I didn't think I needed it. Now I see I do. I call up the pharmacy to have the drug sent over. Even with the Tylenol my breast feels as if I have been stabbed. I call up my mother, because I know she is scared. I know I should talk to my brothers, who by this time have probably had thirteen conversations with Ma, but I am too tired. I go to bed, exhausted, wanting to be taken care of. I think of my grandmother Wadler, round, warm, and cushiony, the one member of the family who thought I was perfect just as I was, and wish she was still around. I think about Nick, who has said he will get out of work as soon as he can and pick up supper, and wonder what is keeping him. He calls, eventually, from the street near his bar. The bank must have messed up, he says, he can't get any money out of the machine; he's got maybe three dollars. I go to meet him at Balducci's market, bumping into Sigmund Freud on the way. "You understand the message he iss sending you," he says. "You vill not depend on him for *nossing*." I banish him from my consciousness by taking him to the deli department and giving him a number and telling him to pick up some derma. There is no derma in Balducci's. By the time he figures it out, I'll have lost him.

When Nick and I get back to my place, just on a point of pride, I set the record straight.

"I'm still the same person I was yesterday, " I tell him. "If we break up every three weeks, we break up every three weeks. I don't want you to treat me any differently."

Which, as it turns out, is the stupidest thing I will say in the course of this whole illness.

And also, as far as Nick is concerned, the least necessary.

IV

IF THIS WERE ANCIENT EGYPT, WHERE PEOPLE WERE BURIED with the things they used most often, the executors of my estate would have no problem making a decision: They would plant me with a phone in one hand and a Diet Pepsi in the other and if it turned out there was a life after death, I would be on the phone, talking to one of my girlfriends or having an emergency session with my shrink. It being late, when I am prone to anxiety attacks, I would probably get an answering machine.

"It's Joyce. It isn't a question of life and death—well, actually, I guess it is, but I mean I can handle it. Um, anyway, this death thing has turned out to be a little more stressful than I thought, and if you have some time, can you give me a call? I mean, if it's not inconvenient. Otherwise, I'll see you the regular time Thursday. One good thing about this: you won't have any trouble getting me to lie down."

But when I get a diagnosis of cancer, it changes. It isn't just that I am numb from the news and the surgery the first day. It isn't even that I need to be alone to sort all this stuff out. I have spent a lifetime sorting things out with my friends. But now, I feel, I am under serious attack, and when the Scud missiles are raining on your head, you don't have time to get on the phone with your girlfriends and say you are terribly depressed. Also, there is something else: I am afraid of negativity. *Cancer* is a scary word: people hear it and think "death," and I don't want that sort of energy around me. I also don't want to hear, however well-meaning, other people's stories. Until now, I thought breast cancer was breast cancer; I had no idea there were different kinds, some more dangerous than others. I also realize that everybody's body is different. I love my friends, I want their support, but hearing a story about a friend of a friend who "had it" and is now doing fine will be a waste of my time. What I need is hard facts about medullary and to educate myself about the options. I'll tell some close friends the diagnosis, but they have to keep it to themselves. Just on a professional level, I don't want this around. Journalists are the biggest gossips in the world and the least reliable—one lunch at Orso's and three hours later word will be all over town that I'm dying, and I'll never sell another book. I'm also making a rule: Information goes out, but unless I ask, it doesn't come in. Herb and I also ask my friends to let me call them. If they want to know the details of what's happening medically, they can call Herb for briefings. Herb calls them Breast Conferences.

Wednesday, the day after the surgery, I get organized. Financially, I'm in good shape. Though living in Manhattan is expensive and my rent is $1,200 a month, my health insurance is paid for by *People* and, after a $1,400 deductible, seems to cover everything. I have $23,000 in my savings account. If worse comes to worse, I can call on my family. It seems a piece of bum luck that I have been diagnosed when I am on an unpaid literary leave, with no money coming in, while if all this had happened two weeks earlier I would be receiving full pay, on sick leave, but it occurs to me that maybe the magazine can change that.

I still have the problem, however, of professional obligations. My publisher has paid a bundle for the M. Butterfly story—"Let's face it, now they own you," Ma had said when I signed the contract—the deadline has already been extended, and I have no idea how long this breast business is going to hang me up. I have the same concern about *People*. I've also promised a magazine editor a piece. My agent and the editor are both out of town, so I can't deal with either the magazine or the book problem; but I make an appointment to go in and talk to the *People* editor, Lanny Jones, the next day. I'm nervous about this. As calm as I'm trying to be, when I have to say the word *cancer* to someone new, I sometimes start crying. I cry easily, and actually, a lot of the time I enjoy it. There is a long-distance phone commercial where a son tells his mama no, nothing is wrong, he's just calling to say he loves her, that dissolves me in thirty seconds. I'm not self-conscious about crying in front of Herb or Nick; when it comes to sobbing in old movies, my macho Italian is usually sniffling along with me, but I feel it would be humiliating to cry in the professional arena. It doesn't go badly, though. I have a few minutes discussing mastectomy where I think I am about to lose it and have to stop talking and have a few sips of coffee, but Lanny is terrific. He agrees to tell no one about my diagnosis and changes my unpaid literary leave to a medical leave—on full pay—and says the resources of the company are behind me. Within two days, four different people from Medical and Benefits have called.

Professional problems out of the way for the moment, I turn to research. I have an advantage: I am a reporter, and so are a lot of my friends. I call up two or three and give them a task: Herb goes to the library and does a hard check on Luke's credentials; Heidi, a magazine editor who I have known for over twenty years, will call the American Cancer Society and the National Institutes of Health; Max, who is the bureau chief for an out-of-town paper, will call his contacts all across the country; we'll all get names for second opinions. There is no way, with a life-threatening disease, I am not getting a second opinion. The reference I put the most stock in comes from an old friend who is a doctor and researcher: "You'll go to Jeanne Petrek at Sloan-Kettering for the surgery; Norton as the oncologist. He's the head of the Breast Cancer Department at Sloan, very sharp. He's a friend, our wives are friends. Make the call and tell him I sent you. No, wait; I'll make the call myself."

It's a relief. But I wonder. What happens to the poor women who don't have medical insurance, and don't have families that can help them, and don't have friends who can pull strings to get them into Sloan-Kettering?

That leaves me with that ongoing problem: Ma. They have an interesting way of dealing with illness in my family. They form little whispering cabals, deciding who can Take It. Or, if they must deliver bad news, they come at you in a roundabout way. "You know your Uncle Murray, in the hospital in Kingston, he's really not doing very well," my Aunt Shirley had told me in a phone conversation years ago. Then she asked to speak to my boyfriend. A few minutes later, he passed back the phone. "Actually," said Shirley, "he's dead."

I never understood this, but now I do: You don't tell the people you love, because you want to protect them. But in doing that, you cut yourself off. I talk to Nick about it. He says mothers are stronger than you think, and anyway, I owe my family the full story. The day after the biopsy, I call her.

"I figured you might be worrying, and I was just wondering if you had any questions," I say.

"Yeah," she says. "What aren't you telling me?"

Trick question. Damn, these mothers are smart. I tell her that there is a small possibility "it" may be in the lymph nodes, but we have no evidence yet of that; and if it is, it's not the end of the road. I tell her that because I am concerned another lump might one day be missed, I am leaning toward mastectomy and reconstruction, but that might not be so bad—I've always thought it would be fun to be able to wear those cute little camisoles, and maybe, at forty-three, I could use a perkier pair.

She's scared. I can tell because she hits me with Second-Generation Wadler Cure-all One: "You know, money is not an issue."

"I know that, Ma," I tell her. "It's okay. I got insurance."

"New underwear, anything cosmetic—that's on me," she says.

"Well, I don't know, Ma," I say. "My bras are very expensive. They run thirty-five, forty-five dollars. I don't know if a poor old widow like you can afford them."

"Thirty-four B is a good size," she says. "I'll bring cash. I'll put a thousand in your account." She starts upping the amount, bargaining with some unseen force. "Three. No, five. Six. Ten. For the things that aren't covered by the insurance—taxis for back and forth to the hospital. New underwear. A wig."

I'm suddenly peeved.

"What makes you think I'm gonna need a wig?" I ask her. "I didn't say anything about chemotherapy. I'm healthy. I *had* cancer. I'm just giving you some remote possibilities, because you asked. Anyway, that stuff about chemotherapy has changed—not everybody loses their hair."

"A blond one," she says. "On me."

V

THIS IS ANOTHER STRANGE THING ABOUT BREAST CANCER: though I have just been told I have a life-threatening disease, it's not like the cold or a flu where you actually feel sick. Physically, the day after the biopsy, I feel as strong as I've ever been. My breast aches, but only mildly, and I can take care of it with the Tylenol. I can't see the cut on my breast when I take off the cotton pads, because it's covered with a row of fancy Band-Aids, but my left breast, despite the amount of tissue that's been removed, looks the same size as the right, and somehow I knew it would. Medically, however, we're all still very confused. NIH doesn't know of any medullary experts. Also, we don't understand why you would do a mastectomy at the same time as the lymph-node surgery. If the lymph-node surgery is to see if the cancer has spread, wouldn't you do that first? If it has spread, why would you take off a breast?

I go back to Barnes & Noble and plunk down the $129 for my old pal, *Breast Cancer, Conservative and Reconstructive Surgery*. I also pick up *The Pill Book: The Illus-*

trated Guide to the Most Prescribed Drugs in the United States, so I will know what they're giving me in the hospital, and one or two paperbacks on breast cancer and a book by Norman Cousins, the former editor of *Saturday Review: Head First: The Biology of Hope and the Healing Power of the Human Spirit.* I remember hearing about Cousins's work a few years ago; he had a serious illness and cured himself by laughing. Thursday evening, before going to Luke's, I start reading the medical books. What they say is a lot stronger than Luke:

Cancers are classified in stages, depending on size, whether they are in the nodes, and whether they have spread to other parts of the body. There are four stages, and stage two is not that great: according to one study, the five-year survival rate is 65 percent. Medullary is rare, accounting for perhaps 7 percent of breast cancers; but it can spread, and if it does, it can kill you. The worst kind of breast cancer, accounting for perhaps 2 percent, is inflammatory. The skin is flushed and has a *peau d'orange* texture—exactly what I saw on my breast in the doctor's office the day my lump was discovered. Very few people live beyond five years with inflammatory cancer. I am petrified. I don't care that the lab reports have classified my cancer as medullary. They were just the first reports; what if they made a mistake? And even if it's only medullary, these statistics are hell. I call up Nick, convinced I am doomed, and ask if I can spend the night. "You're driving yourself crazy here," he says. "What do you care what some book says? Maybe it's out of date. You know your doctor says you have the best kind." I am not interested in anything Nick has to say. I just want to be next to him. I take a cab up to his place and in bed burrow my head into the nook of his neck, pressing as close to him as I can.

At nine the next morning, as Nick goes off to work, I meet Herb at Dr. Luke's. My breast, when Luke takes off the Band-Aids and pulls out the sutures, has a thick pink scar, but considering the way he was tunneling around in there, I think I heal great. The problem is, I'm so frightened by what I've read in the medical books, I'm almost stuttering. When I tell Luke about my research, he is not happy. He knows some patients do this—lawyers, usually—but it's not a great thing to do he says, if you're not a doctor, because you can easily misinterpret things. I do *not* have inflammatory cancer. It is true that based on size I have a stage-two cancer, but medullary is not the average breast cancer. I have, he repeats, a very favorable case.

We move on to the big decision: mastectomy or lumpectomy. I still don't understand why one would decide about mastectomy before knowing if cancer has spread and is in the lymph nodes. Luke says one has nothing to do with the other. Lymph-node dissection is diagnostic—it gives you an indication of whether the cancer has spread. Mastectomy or lumpectomy has to do with treating the breast and killing any cancer which might remain. If the cancer had been found in a few places on the breast, a doctor would likely recommend mastectomy. If one is worried about recurrence, one might also.

Herb wants to know the statistics on recurrence. Luke says with lumpectomy it's 15 or 20 percent; with mastectomy, it's down to 4. My chances of getting cancer in the other breast is higher than other people's—7 percent for the next ten years—but Luke does not recommend a prophylactic mastectomy. He's sending me for a mammogram, but he sees no swelling of the lymph nodes under my right arm or any other indication of trouble.

I want to know what reconstruction involves. Luke says at the time of the lymph-node surgery, he'd remove the breast tissue, leave most of the skin, but remove the nipple—it's safer that way, because in one out of four times, the cancer is in the nipple. Then a plastic surgeon would put in an implant and construct a new breast. It will look good on the outside, he stresses, but it won't *feel* like a breast. It's an artificial implant. I try to imagine what it will feel like: a contact lens which at first you are always aware of, then never feel? A football? There is also something that troubles me, that Luke doesn't seem to be taking into consideration: if you opt for mastectomy and come out of surgery to learn that cancer *is* in the lymph nodes, it seems to me it's an awful lot to deal with at once.

I am lost. I ask, since the cure rate is the same with mastectomy and lumpectomy, what the doctor recommends.

"I think mastectomy is the better treatment for you," Luke says. "You've got difficult breasts—large, lumpy—and you're worried about recurrence. Lumpectomy is for people who say, 'I don't want to lose the breast no matter what.' That wasn't your response. The only advantage of lumpectomy is that it preserves the breast. But it's your decision."

It is true, I think, that my first reaction was "Take off the breast"—but that was before I knew what reconstruction involved. Now that I see, I'm not certain. I ask Luke, aside from statistics and my case, if he has a personal bias. He says that he has had three medullary patients, and since one had a recurrence, he leans toward reconstruction. He also says that since he took so much tissue out of the breast, reconstruction will probably give me the better cosmetic result. I tell him I don't think that will be a problem—my breast seems to still be the same size.

"That's swelling from the surgery, and some pockets of air," he says. "When it goes down, it may be much smaller."

He suggests I talk to a plastic surgeon—there is one in particular he thinks would be temperamentally suited for me, because he's an artist as well as a doctor. I take this to mean that Luke is either classifying me among a group of patients who are not so stable and are likely to cut off an ear or that he has been influenced by Herb's beard, but I'm happy to be seeing the artists' doctor. Maybe when we get to his office, he'll offer us an espresso. I haven't had any breakfast. I could use it.

My mammogram, which we have taken across the street, is normal, except for what the report calls "a large radiolucency, in the left breast, consistent with residual air." Apparently, Luke is right: my nice plump breast is pumped up like a Macy's balloon and may deflate at any moment. I have a sudden, crazy image of me on a date and a fellow reaching over to cop a high-school kind of feel, when suddenly, "Pffffooooot"—meltdown.

Then, in what's turning into a cancer triathlon, Herb and I rush twenty blocks to the office of the plastic surgeon, Dr. Frank Veteran, in the Eighties, off Fifth. I'm a little worried about Herb; he's the sort of man who feels uncomfortable in the lingerie department of Saks. I'm remembering some photos of mastectomy from my medical books and wondering how graphic this consultation is going to get. But at the same time I'm excited. In the taxi, I have come up with a wonderful idea: rather than mastectomy and reconstruction, why not, after treating my breast with radiation, do a reduction? If I get rid of, say, 30 percent of breast, I remove 30 percent of potentially dangerous cancer-bearing tissue. I won't have to run around nippleless or with a football in my chest. I could also end up with a very pretty pair of breasts. I do like my body, basically; there are times I look at myself naked and think I'm gorgeous, but as I've gotten older, or have seen skinny women with high little breasts at the gym, I have sometimes felt bad, looking at my sag, and wondered what it would be like to have a lift.

I like Dr. Veteran, too. He's not slick. There's an air about him that suggests he has had personal experience with serious illness. Now, after Dr. Veteran examines me, I hit him with my idea. It's original all right—Veteran doesn't know of anyone who's done it—but he also says it's not a good idea. Radiated tissue is difficult to work with; some of the smaller blood vessels are destroyed; it doesn't heal as well as normal skin. If one must operate on radiated tissue in order to save a life, one does, but as elective surgery, he would prefer not. Doing the reduction *before* the radiation, he says, is not a good idea either. Radiation can affect breast size: some people get as much as a cup larger or smaller, and you might end up with two different-sized breasts. More importantly, reduction is major surgery, which involves aftereffects Dr. Veteran considers foolhardy for cancer patients. There is a great deal of internal scarring, which can interfere with getting a good picture on a mammogram. That internal scarring also reduces the blood flow to the breast, often resulting in patches of fat necrosis, or dead fat cells. In themselves they are not usually problems, but they can appear on a mammogram as lumps, causing diagnostic confusion. I already have a long scar from my lumpectomy, which could further reduce blood flow. Finally, a breast reduction takes time to heal, and that could delay the time before which I begin radiation treatment. This is cancer; the medical considerations have to come first. My skin is good; I'm young; I can get "a very good cosmetic result" with reconstruction. The words "very good cosmetic result" disturb me. Is it a suggestion that I really could use a new pair? Is the doctor saying, in a roundabout way, that what he has seen in the examining room is awful? I picture Joan Rivers, in an off-camera booth, feeding the doctor lines: "She takes off her bra," she says, "she could nurse Soho."

Reduction dismissed as an alternative, the doctor explains reconstruction: At the time of the mastectomy, working with Luke, he would put an expander, made of silicone, under the muscles of my chest. You couldn't put it directly under the skin, as you would with breast augmentation, because all the breast tissue is gone, and there would be nothing to serve as a cushion between the implant and the skin. Over a four- to six-week period, depending on how large the new breast was going to be, a saline solution would be injected into the implant, enlarging it. The muscles on top of the implant would stretch and expand, just as they do in pregnancy—but just as in pregnancy, one couldn't stretch them all at once. After two or three months, after the tissue around the implant had "settled down," there would be a second operation, and a permanent prosthesis replaces the expander. If I was having chemotherapy, I would have to wait a longer period of time before surgery, because chemotherapy usually brings down the white blood cell count, increasing the risk of infection. The usual course of chemotherapy is six months. Finally, in the case of large breasted women like myself, there would be a third operation, a reduction on the healthy breast, to make it match the first. At that time, the surgeon would build a nipple for the reconstructed breast. Again, there would be a waiting period—at least a month—to make sure the swelling of the reconstructed breast had gone down and you were getting a good "match." Years ago, surgeons sometimes tried to save the nipple after removing it by attaching it temporarily to another area of the body and then reattaching it, but the results were not very good— the nipple usually lost pigmentation and looked like a raisin, the doctor says. He prefers nipple "sharing"— grafting half the nipple from the opposite breast. He can also fashion a nipple from a skin graft, usually taken from near the crease of the groin, which hides the scar. He tattoos an areola.

As somebody who is terrified of general anesthesia, this is awful—I'm now looking at three extra operations, not one. Then the doctor shows us the pictures and it's worse: a color Polaroid of a woman whose breast looks like a halved grapefruit. The shape is perfectly round and unnatural; a thick red scar runs from one side to the other; she has no nipple and no areola.

"I can't walk around for six months looking like that," I say. "It's like a nuclear catastrophe."

Then I feel terrible. I am talking to an artist about his

work, and it is probably just the first step, after the insert has been pumped up.

"What I mean is, it just sort of throws me—the idea of walking around like that with no nipple. I'm sure when it's all finished it looks really nice," I say.

The doctor shows us more Polaroids, including women with their finished breasts, who look much better. He says there are implants he can use for a more natural look; that while every implant feels the same, all breast tissue is different, so that, when they are touched, my breasts may not feel the same. His patients tell him, however, that after a while they are not aware of the implant—it just becomes their breast. He's a lovely guy: It's running on two-thirty; we were booked at the last minute; I'm sure he hasn't had any lunch. But he acts like he has all the time in the world to answer our questions.

"Is there anything else you're wondering about?" he asks, finally.

I've got one last question, very important: "You know any good French restaurants in the neighborhood?"

He doesn't just give us the name; he makes the reservation. We go to lunch, taking solace in onion soup. I like this doctor, I tell Herb. But unless I learn mastectomy is essential for my health, having seen what reconstruction involves, the process is out—there is no way I am going to do those things to my body.

I also think of something else.

"You know how we're always saying we miss things," I say to Herb. "We weren't around for Paris in the twenties; we weren't reporters in New York in the forties; I had tickets to Woodstock—too much mud; I didn't go. It just hit me, all these stories we've been seeing about breast cancer—for this trend, I'm right on time."

VI

SATURDAY, FOUR DAYS AFTER MY DIAGNOSIS, I WAKE UP WITH
a nightmare: My assistant, Stéphane, and I are in France,
driving in my father's car, a big Chevy of some sort, in a
part of the country that is new to us. The people are suspicious of us and not friendly, and the terrain is very
strange: ditches of water, irregularly shaped little lakes,
some covered with ice. I don't know if Stéphane or I am
driving; I only know that we have to be careful. Then,
suddenly, we are on a lake. At first we are okay, driving
on top of the water, and then we start to sink. I am trying
to figure out how to get out and still save my father's car,
which is fairly new and expensive: Should we roll the
windows shut, so it doesn't sink as fast? But if we do that,
and the doors stick, we'll be trapped. So maybe we
should just forget the car and get out. Somehow, as the
car sinks, we do get out, but I am left in strange country
without anything. I am supposed to be taking care of Stéphane—he is younger than me and my responsibility—
but suddenly I have no money. I am more dependent
than ever on Stéph in this strange territory, and I am

thinking that my father's car is sitting at the bottom of this lake and he will blame me. Then I wake up, and instead of reality being better, it is worse:

Oh shit, I have cancer. Excuse me, that is a negative thought; cancel it. I *had* cancer. I *had* a cancer in my breast. Now it is out.

I am trying to be exceptionally positive because some of the cancer books I've been collecting claim that cancer cells are always popping up in people; the average person may "get" cancer seven times a year, but a healthy immune system knocks them out. Some writers, including Cousins, have this theory, which normally I would consider crackpot, that stress literally weakens the immune system, while positive energy and laughter create, uh, endorphins or something that helps the immune system battle the disease—so don't worry, be happy. But how can you be happy when, according to some of these books, by the time a cancerous lump is big enough to be felt—around one centimeter—it contains one billion cells and has been in your body ten years, and chances are you've got millions of cancer cells sloshing through your bloodstream, looking to own, not rent?

"Yes, we *were* very happy in Miss Wadler's left breast for a long time. It was a wonderful space. You've seen it in a T-shirt—it's enormous. But now, the family is growing, and we're looking for something with a little more air and light—like maybe her lungs and the top of her head."

If there's a chance positive thinking can work, I feel I should try it, but I am skeptical. If being a worrier has contributed to this disease, am I going to be able to alter my personality quickly enough to stop it? I've had fifteen years of therapy just trying to convince myself I am lovable enough for some man to want to marry me. My shrink and I have been slogging back and forth over this terrain so often that I now see us locked into a primitive and simpleminded dialogue, like some floundering psychoanalytic Tarzan and Jane: "Hello, me Joyce, me worthless." "No, you not worthless, you Joyce." Years of this stuff and I still haven't been able to pull off the one space I really want in American journalism: the *New York Times* wedding page.

"For bachelors and criminals, Sundays are bad," I had said to Bernard, one gray afternoon in Paris, when we walked through the deserted streets of a family neighborhood in the Nineteenth Arrondissement, and the world seemed shuttered closed around us.

Today is a Saturday, but it seems equally grim: I can't call doctors. Herb is spending the day with a buddy in Brooklyn, which is good—I want him to have some time off. I'm still not sure how to deal with cancer with my friends. There's no word from Nick, so I assume he is planning to see The Magnificent Obsession or brooding about the fact that he is not. This relationship, I think, is really lunatic; if one of us had a maid or a butler, we could do a remake of *La Ronde*. I feel bleak. Getting up and going for breakfast at the Greek coffee shop, I try to distract myself with the papers, but I cannot. As I read the *Times,* a fat tear plops on the page. Looking up, I see Sammy, the counter man, staring at me, wondering what is wrong.

"I have cancer—I *had* cancer," I want to tell him, but I can't, because that is not a positive thought.

Instead, I go home and busy myself with everything-here-is-normal, life-affirming acts. I pay my bills. I write a thank-you note to the Time, Inc., doctor who got me to a specialist so quickly, which makes me think of the joke about the first thing a debutante does after an orgy. (Writes thirty-five thank-you notes.) I take my expensive medical book back to Barnes & Noble and ask if I can get my $129 back. No problem. Great. Maybe they have a branch where I can give back my cancer. Then I hit Daffy's, a discount clothing store, across the street. I am going to an Oscar party with Nick on Monday, and I want something new and pretty. They're blasting the sound track from *Oklahoma* in the store, which makes me feel better in a manic sort of way. I love show tunes. I took a whole bunch with me to Paris, and when I got scared and had to do an interview with a fancy diplomat, I used to psych myself up with *Guys and Dolls*. By the end of my first hitch, my French was good enough that every once in a while I could sing the first verse of "I got the horse right here," to my newsstand dealer, who always had his nose stuck in the racing form. Now, hopped up on Hammerstein and forcing myself into a future-positive mode, I grab an armload of summer clothes and find myself in the dressing room with two strapless, low-cut dresses unlike anything I have ever owned in my life: a lime green fifties number that looks like something Audrey Hepburn would have brought back from Paris in *Sabrina,* and a short black sheath with gold beading. Both show more cleavage than I show at the beach, which is fine with me: Norman Cousins says defiance is good for disease—I'll show you defiance. I don't like the dresses on me at all, and I realize it's a good thing, because I now have a new problem when shopping: What size are my breasts going to be this summer? Is the left one even going to *be* there? My solution is buying a loose, striped blue-and-white blouse—very Oxford rowing team—and a straw boater.

They look so breezy and summery and dapper, like the young Maurice Chevalier in *One Hour with You*. Cancer couldn't get Maurice Chevalier.

But I am still scared. Sad, too. Getting home with my new clothes, I check my answering machine, hoping for a message from Nick. There is none. It is still early, not even noon, and possibly, as is his pattern, he will call in a few hours, telling me he is making a red sauce, asking me if I'd like to come up and share it. It is not a very flattering invitation, coming as it does last minute. I would really like to be seeing a man who thought I was valuable enough to book a little earlier in the week, but I am not so confident with the opposite sex as Nick. Discounting a short affair at the end of my last stay in Paris, I had been four years without a boyfriend before I started seeing him, during which time the credo of Greenwich Village women had gone from "A woman without a man is like a fish without a bicycle" to "A woman over forty has a better chance of being killed by a terrorist than marrying." Five months into my first hitch in France, dating like crazy but unable to get anything off the ground, it had reached a point where even Bernard, who had made the most notorious sexual error in the history of the planet, was stumped.

"We are all wondering, Joyce," he said, one perfect July day, as we were sitting out front at The Select, "how is it you can be alone in Paris?"

"Listen, Bernard," I said, "you proposed to somebody who shaves, and you're telling me *I* got problems with relationships?"

Nick always had a girl. He had told me stories about his adventures when we first started dating—crazy, outrageous stories in which he was always the passive party: a rape complainant he had met down at criminal court, who made love to him in the press room; a lesbian, apparently conflicted, who took out his penis in a bar; a feminist writer, back in the seventies, who told him she wouldn't mind sleeping with him but wanted to make sure that he wasn't "anybody else's."

"I'll tell you how it is," Nick had said. "I'm married to one, I'm in love with another one, and I'm living with a third one."

"C'mon home," the woman said.

I knew Nick could not be so passive as he suggested: a woman does not put her hand on a man's penis unless she has been given very strong encouragement. I had also started to see a pattern in his love affairs I did not like at all: the women who cared for Nick, some of whom sounded terrific, he always threw over for women he loved passionately and who treated him as badly as he treats me. He seemed aware of it, too.

"I always throw the good ones away," he told me, a few days before the weekend he had gone off with his old girl.

And yet, breaking up with Nick is something I cannot do. I have seen him standing outside the two-star restaurant where his son works as a waiter and apprentice chef, staring at him through the window. "There he is—what a good looking kid. God, I love my son," he said. He has told me that no, in his two marriages, he did not get up in the morning and turn on television; he doted on his wives. If he ignores me, it therefore follows, it must somehow be my fault, for certainly Nick can love.

I feel myself getting more depressed and try to think of the best way to fight it. I do have two girlfriends who had breast cancer and are fine. I could talk to them, but I'm not sure that would make me feel better: they both had tumors the size of peas. It's scaring me to be the girl with the biggest one on the block. It would be great, tonight, to go put on some high heels and go dancing—the old Catskills cha-cha solution—get as far away from cancer as I can, but I can't think of anyone to ask. I decide to keep shopping. What I really need, it occurs to me, is an art deco martini shaker. I do not cook; I rarely entertain; I never had a martini until the night Nick took me to the Rainbow Room. But now, with cancer at my tail, I envision a new life in which I will have people over for drinks and wear a thirties gown cut on the bias, and my apartment will not be cluttered with books and computer discs and bikini underpants drying on the shower-curtain rod, but will resemble something in a Fred Astaire movie. I will stand off to the side, with a martini glass in my hand and three suitors around me, and whatever they say, I will laugh musically—"Ahahaha." This is probably what I have been doing wrong with guys all these years: I haven't laughed musically.

Giddy with the stylish new life I have created for myself, I rush back down to the street. But the high is speedy and laced with too much anxiety to last. Walking west through the Village to Greenwich Avenue, the terror muscles its way to the top, and I have the same awful feeling I had the day I discovered my lump: someone has pushed a fast-forward button, and much sooner than expected, I am going to die. Only now that fear is fact. I think about how, as Paris became an old friend, I thought there would be a time I would live there, and now I won't. I think about how Herb and I, when we pass the Village Nursing Home on Hudson Street, say, yeah, that's where we'll end up. I feel cursed—why the hell did this have to happen to me?—and alone. People have said call anytime, but I'm facing death, not a three-pound weight gain or trouble with a boss, who can understand it who hasn't been there? Crossing Seventh Avenue, I start to cry in the street. I keep shopping anyway. I find a beautiful stainless steel art deco shaker, wondering how much time I'm going to have to use it. Then, feeling my positive thinking is floundering, I try to remember advice from my cancer books. Nutrition, they say, is important. I go to the supermarket and push my cart up and down the aisles, searching for foods which are particularly healthy. I study the Pepperidge Farm breads for a long time. What's potentially more life-saving? Whole Wheat? Crunchy Granola? Raisin Bran? If breast cancer really is on the rise they should introduce a new line: Raisin Lump. No, I haven't heard one thing associating raisins with cancer prevention. Wait, I've got it: MammoGran.

Then, because according to Norman Cousins a former director of Sloan-Kettering has said zinc is good for fighting cancer, I go to a health-food store to get zinc. I hate health-food stores. The combination of sitar music and incense and Transcendental Meditation posters makes me want to give someone a smack. My brother Martin, for a while, was a follower of Maharishi Mahesh

Yogi. He taught TM at a wage so low he could not afford a winter coat, while the Maharishi flew around in a private jet and he convinced everybody in the family to meditate, telling them it would reduce their chance of heart attack. There is practically nothing the people in my family will not do if you tell them it will reduce their chance of heart attack. Grandma meditated also. She kept a picture of Martin and the Maharishi on the coffee table and called the Maharishi, with his long white beard, Martin's "rebbe." Martin said meditating brought down Grandma's blood pressure, but I never believed him and tried to subvert him by trying to get Gram to tell me her mantra, which she never would.

Now I have cancer and am prepared to explore the wisdom of Eastern ways. I get a basket from the checkout girl, who has apparently seen through me with her invisible third eye and gives me a chilly look. I zap back a message on Telepathic Express.

"In my previous life, I was Mahatma Gandhi," I tell her. "All I can say about this incarnation is, somebody screwed up big. Could you believe, the father of India with knockers in a forty-five-dollar Wacoal brassiere?— though I gotta say, I do look kind of cute. Anyway, what I wanted to tell you—the way this woman eats, you wouldn't believe. A package of Hershey's kisses is her idea of a healthy midmorning snack—the little packs, fifty-five cents, eight kisses; you know the ones I mean? No, of course, you don't. My earthly bod—I'm dying in here. Please help this dame out. Get her some tofu snaps or something. I love your pallor, by the way. You sure we didn't get it on in a previous life in Bangladesh?"

I go home, exhausted, and look over the day's purchases: a striped blouse and a straw boater, suitable for a remake of *Gigi*; a martini mixer for a drink I have no idea how to make; two thousand tablets each of zinc and vitamin B and vitamin C. The way this is going, I think, next thing you know I'll be boarding the Steve McQueen flight to Mexico and sucking on peach pits. The time has come to call a friend. I choose Jane, a psychotherapist, who had cancer six years ago. She and her husband are just leaving town, so Jane can't talk long, but she gives me a number where she can be reached later in the weekend and another for a breast cancer support group called SHARE. I call SHARE. A machine answers. I leave a message.

Then, last minute as usual, I hear from Nick, and we get into the old my-place-or-yours debate.

"You don't want me to come down just because you're sick?" he says.

"I'm *not* sick," I shoot back.

Manipulative little prick. It's actually pretty deft: I

got cancer; he's using it to get what he wants. Except, the truth is, I prefer Nick's place: he's got the movies; he's got food in the house; his son lives with him, and he's a lovely kid. It's only because of the cancer, I want Nick to come to me, to show me he's willing to baby me. I am, I decide, completely nuts. Of course, Nick is too. We continue to negotiate, wanting the same thing, but needing to let the other know we are not easy, and finally settling on a deal: he'll pay my cab fare and make supper; I'll bring the martinis. I fuss before going uptown, because I don't want to look like a sick person. I want to look great. I smear single girl gunk all over my body and put on black stretch pants and a blue silk shirt. I knot a scarf around my neck like a French girl and put on some very delicate silver Victorian bracelets. I like making love to Nick absolutely naked except for earrings and nail polish and two wrists of bracelets. When I get uptown, Nick opens the door all in white, with a black bow tie, and a dishtowel over his arm.

"I got dressed like a waiter," he says. "How many of your boyfriends have ever done that for you?"

We have a perfect time: catch the end of the Knicks game, have supper, watch *Woman of the Year,* cry at the part where Katharine Hepburn realizes what a botch she's made of her marriage, and make love. I feel good. The cancer skirts around the edge of my consciousness; but enjoying Nick, I can put it out of my mind.

Sunday evening, after I've gone home to let Nick catch up on work, a volunteer from SHARE calls. The organization, she explains, does not recommend doctors, nor does she know any medullary cancer specialists. She does, however, give me the name of medical libraries and research groups, and says she'll be happy to answer any questions. Despite my reading, I have a lot: What are the effects of lymph-node surgery on your arm? What does radiation feel like? What really happens when you have chemotherapy—do you throw up all the time?

The volunteer, who is my age and single, talks to me as if we are friends. Lymph-node removal is serious surgery, she says, I will be able to type and use my arm, but most people don't have full range of motion for a few weeks. Something like pulling a sweater over my head might be difficult. She had cancer four years ago and was treated with lumpectomy and radiation. This year, she had a recurrence. Because a breast cannot be radiated twice, she had a mastectomy. She plans to have a reconstruction, but after radiation a simple implant may fail, and doctors then may have to do a far more complicated procedure in which they graft muscle and tissue from her back to her chest. I start getting nervous. Nobody told me you couldn't radiate a breast twice; it makes my decision about whether to have lumpectomy or mastectomy even more complicated.

The volunteer continues: Since 1988, she says, because of the findings of the National Cancer Institute, most breast-cancer patients have some form of chemotherapy, even if cancer is not in the lymph nodes. There are two combinations of drugs that are commonly used: CMF, which is Cytoxan, methotrexate, and 5 fluorouracil; or CAF, which is Cytoxan, Adriamycin, and 5 fluorouracil. If you receive CMF, you may not lose your hair; if you get CAF, which is stronger, you definitely will. You may also have other problems: nausea, skin rash, exhaustion, low-level infections, early menopause. She is now taking CAF and often has mouth sores and vaginal infections, and is frequently nauseous and weak. Some days are good, some days are bad. When she first was diagnosed, she lived with a man; but now she lives alone, and that is hard. Friends have difficulty understanding. They seem to think that when surgery is over, treatment is over, and it is not. When she needs support now, she goes either to her mother or to other members of SHARE. Being with a group of people who have had similar experiences is very comforting.

I am having the opposite experience: the more this

woman talks, the more upset I become. Some of the nicest times I have had with Nick were on the beach. Soon after we started dating, we went out to Montauk and splurged on a room with a private deck overlooking the ocean. I sunned topless, in a big hat and shades, and half-dozing, looked over at Nick and saw him staring at me. "God, you look fantastic," he said. Our first morning together, when I was showering, he had pulled back the curtains. "Look at this voluptuous woman in my shower—I can't believe it; I ought to get down on my knees and thank God," he said, and stepped in. Now I am picturing the good times disappearing. I see myself with one breast and sores on my mouth, too ill to even take care of myself. I see a club to which I do not want to belong and yet have been drafted—a fellowship of sick people.

I get off the phone with the volunteer and call up Nick. Twenty minutes later, I'm up at his place, telling him everything the volunteer has told me. He sits me down on his bed and does his bad cop act. I think it's an act, anyway. He's never been this tough.

"You know what you're doing? You're making yourself crazy again," he says. "I'm not going to let you do that to yourself. You don't know any of that stuff is going to happen to you. What chance did your doctor say there was of this cancer being anywhere else in your body?

Small, very small. This is gonna turn out to be nothing. A year from now, you're gonna be telling me I was right."

He suggests a movie to get my mind off it. I opt for "The Singing Detective," a Masterpiece Theater Playhouse thing I hear is good. Nick gets me a glass of wine, and a T-shirt to sleep in, and we lie back in bed, and I settle in on his chest. The film opens with a scene in a British hospital ward. The patients are crippled and deranged. Suddenly I am sobbing so violently my body is shaking. Nick clicks off the movie and puts his arms around me.

"Baby, what's going on?" he says. "Is it going to be like this forever?"

"I don't know," I say.

VII

IT'S A RELIEF, ON MONDAY, TO BE ABLE TO GET BACK TO RE-search. The only thing is, I am finding a new problem: I am dealing with a growing group of specialists—a breast surgeon, plastic surgeon, oncologist, radiologist. Each specialist puts his field first and is somewhat ignorant—at times even disdainful—of the others. The cancer surgeons, when they discuss reduction surgery—an idea I haven't dismissed—seem to regard it as a hideous, even frivolous, procedure. Dr. Luke, when I talk things over with him after seeing Dr. Veteran, suggests doing a reduction *after* I'm done with lumpectomy and radiation; he isn't aware plastic surgeons have difficulty working with irradiated tissue. Even if I give up my idea of reduction, there will be three to four people involved.

"I understand that I don't see the oncologist until after the lymph-node surgery, and the radiation doctor comes in after that," I tell a nursing assistant at Sloan-Kettering, when I make an appointment. "But who's in charge?"

"There will be a group of doctors, who will all be

monitoring you along the way," she says cheerfully, "but as far as who's in charge—in a sense, you are."

In a sense, that's good—I should be the one to have the final say about what happens to my body. In another, it's terrifying. I know nothing about science; I'm one of those people who's still not sure what makes planes stay up. What this disease needs, I decide, is a contractor—or at least a place where we could get all the specialists in one room.

On the positive side, it turns out that while the United States is lousy on health care, we are a great nation for booklets. Call 1–800–4–CANCER, the Cancer Information Service at the National Cancer Institute, and you can speak to a cancer expert, get fact sheets, and order pamphlets on everything from treatment to psychological support. They have a service called Physician's Data Query, or PDQ, which sends information on cancer treatment to patients and their doctors, so that even if you live in Podunk, you can still get up-to-date information on what's happening.

I also get a lot of information from the American Cancer Society's Cancer Response System, at 1–800–ACS–2345. Their fact sheet, which, like NCI's, is reviewed and updated every few months, contains the best news I've gotten since my diagnosis: "Medullary carcinoma accounts for about 7 percent of breast cancers. It seems to grow in a capsule within the duct, and although it can become quite large, it does not metastasize as frequently as others and has a better outlook." For the first time since Dr. Luke told me the lump was malignant, I have a deep sense of relief: this is not just one doctor snowing me.

I also have good news, midweek, on the professional front: My publisher says not to worry about the deadline for my book, just concentrate on my health. The magazine editor whom I've promised a piece not only says the same but adds something that cheers me.

"I'll tell you a secret," she says. "I've got leukemia—chronic lymphocytic. It's supposed to be the best kind. Nobody here knows. I found out during my last job, when I had a physical and they found my white blood counts were really low."

She's the last person I'd think has cancer—a beautiful woman in her late fifties who takes manuscripts home and still makes time to play tennis and go skiing.

"You just got back from Vail," I say.

"Yeah," she says. "Statistically, I'm supposed to be dead. The median survival time for this kind of leukemia is six years. But I've got this theory. I think they're making so many advances with cancer so fast that by the time they get around to publishing the stats, they're five years old."

I'm touched that this woman, with whom I have mainly a professional relationship, has told me her story. But what affects me more is the realization that there are probably a lot of people like her all around me: a secret society of cancer survivors, whom no one is aware of because of the stigma of the disease.

Meanwhile, I'm beat. I run around town, picking up medical records and my last four years of mammograms from the Guttman Institute. The mammograms are important to me. I'm hoping someone will be able to spot the tumor that was missed a year ago and use it to find any other dangerous lumps that may exist. There is one thing which may make this difficult: I do not have a mammogram of my breast from the time I discovered my malignant lump. I had asked Luke if one should be taken on my second visit, when he said I would need a biopsy, and he had said it would not be a good idea: the lump would throw a shadow on the breast tissue; it would be better to take a mammogram after it came out. I thought a record might be helpful, but I said nothing—Luke was the doctor. Now I am sorry I didn't speak up.

I'm also not happy with Luke when I get a copy of the aspiration lab report. The results are a lot more ominous than Luke told me in our phone conversation: "Few individual and many clusters of markedly atypical cells in an acute inflammatory and necrotic background," the report reads in part. "The epithelial atypia is highly suspicious for malignancy. . . ." It is possible Luke's paternalism extends beyond an arm thrown warmly around one's shoulder. If so, or if he's not going to give me all the facts, he's not the doctor for me.

I call back the Time, Inc., doctor to talk some more about second opinions. He explains that when looking for a second opinion, it is best to look for a doctor who has not been trained at the same institute as your first one—that way, you are more likely to get a fresh point of view. When I tell him that I am planning to see Dr. Norton at Sloan-Kettering, he is impressed, but cautionary, telling me Norton is not the easiest doctor to get in to see. I explain he's the friend of a friend.

"It's a little gauche," the doctor says, "but I suppose if it works. . . ."

Gauche? My life is on the line and this guy is talking like I've violated Miss Manners' Guide to Malignancies?

"Listen," I say, "I've used connections to get interviews with movie stars. You think I'm not going to do everything I can when I'm fighting for my life?"

I have also remembered something about the Guttman that disturbs me—something so important it's hard for me to believe it slipped my mind: Last year, after I had my mammogram and had been examined by a doctor, a second doctor was called in to check out a suspicious lump. That had never happened before. I could not swear the lump was the one which ultimately proved malignant; I am not even 100 percent sure it was in the left breast. I just remember the second doctor saying the words I always heard: "This is nothing." Now I'm angry. If medullary cancer accounts for 7 percent of breast cancers, shouldn't the doctors be aware of its ability to masquerade as a benign lump? Aspiration is a two-minute procedure. If my lump was suspicious enough to warrant a second doctor, why didn't someone suggest it?

I'm also having a lot of difficulty making up my mind about whether or not to have a mastectomy and reconstruction. I had felt certain Friday, when Herb and I looked at the pictures, but early in the week Dr. Veteran, thinking about my fear of surgery, calls with a way to reduce the number of operations from three to two: rather than use an expander, which will later be replaced with an implant, he can use something called the Becker Expander, which will remain inside the body. It sounds good, but the shape I will have if we use this device— which the doctor himself describes as "grapefruit"—does not. My breasts may not be saluting the sun, but they have their charm, and I am not about to replace them with a set of citrus. I can't believe that I'm the only woman in America who's had the idea of treating cancer with lumpectomy and reduction, either. I continue reporting. I call the American College of Radiologists and the American Society of Plastic and Reconstructive Surgeons. I hear of no one who has done reduction and lumpectomy to treat and prevent the disease.

I read. Despite Dr. Luke's warnings that I may misinterpret information, discarding research is an idea I've discarded. It's my body and my life. I read about drugs; I read about nutrition; I read about alternative therapies like visualization, where you are supposed to picture cancer cells in your body and tell them to drop dead. NCI has included in its freebie pack a book called *Fighting Cancer*, by Richard Block, the cofounder of the H & R Block income tax company. In 1978, Block had been told he had inoperable lung cancer and was doomed. Two years later, he was cured. He advocates medical treatment combined with positive thinking and is convinced stress contributes to the disease: "Chronic depression and stress depress the immune response," he writes. "It has been demonstrated that tumors grow faster in mice under stress." I wonder how you give a lady mouse stress. Tell her she's had three too many litters and won't be made partner? Block, anyway, has an affirmation to be read out loud daily, a life-is-swell statement that is so icky-gooey that I want to hide it, perhaps under cover of one of Anaïs Nin's dirty books. Reading the affirmation out loud, I feel like a jerk. But Block is alive and publishing, and a former director of the National Cancer Institute, Dr. Vincent DeVita, wrote the introduction. I keep the book on my bedside table and at night, after looking around the room to make sure nobody has snuck in the apartment and can see me, read the affirmation, trying to shut out the cynical voices running counterpoint against them.

"I realize negative thoughts create negative experiences and positive thoughts create positive experiences," I say. "Therefore I now decide to control my thoughts and think of the positive good side of me and my world."

"Oh, yeah?" the negative voice says. "Quick, tell me the positive good side of genocide. I'm dying to hear it."

I continue:

"I realize the spoken word is the most powerful. Therefore I speak good thoughts out loud and count my blessings out loud daily. I focus my thought energy on the good of me, of you, of today, of life."

"You know how this makes me focus *my* thought energy?" a slightly accented voice says. "Like I had one too many Sacher tortes and I'm gonna throw up."

"That me or you?" I ask.

"It's me," says Freud, making himself at home in a corner armchair. "That vas a rotten stunt you pulled in Balducci's the other veek, by the vay. Throwing me over for the Saint of the Perpetual Hard-on. Now I find you reading this. Turn off your negative thoughts. Do you think you can get away from the unconscious just like that? Never underestimate the power of the unconscious. It paid for a lot of summer houses on the Cape."

"Beat it, Sigmund," I tell him. "You're giving me stress."

What I really am beginning to believe, as I stay up nights reading, is that this stress thing, which I have been trying so hard to control, has gotten a little out of hand. Stress may, for all I know, depress the immune system, but the theory that insecure, self-critical people who put the needs of others before their own are prone to the disease strikes me as nonsense. There are an awful lot of insecure, self-critical people I know who do not have cancer. But it's a hard theory to beat down when there is so much of it around. There's a best-seller called *Love*,

Medicine, and Miracles by Dr. Bernie Siegel, a surgeon who teaches at Yale, that takes that view. Siegel also writes, "Women who have unhappy love relationships are especially prone to breast and cervical cancers" and demands patients ask themselves, "Why did you need this illness?" It infuriates me. Though I grew up in a house where my grandmother, if she dropped a book, kissed it when she picked it up from the floor, I throw this book on the floor, stomp on it, and throw it out. "Why do I need this book?" I say. And yet I can't shake Siegel's theory entirely, because a small part of me worries that he has a point. Is it possible that if you constantly beat yourself up, holding yourself up to impossible standards, figuratively eating away at yourself, that the body follows through? Who tore at himself with worry more than my father? How much pleasure was he ever able to have in life? How much fun was it for me, those first few months in Paris, when I was trying to operate as a reporter and didn't know enough French to leave a message asking somebody to return a call?

My mother seems to be thinking along the same lines.

"You think maybe the reason this happened is the book and all that time you spent in France?" Ma says.

———

This only appears to be a question. What it actually is is a statement of fact: "You made yourself sick." I grew up with this, so to a certain extent, I can dismiss it.

"If you're telling me working too hard gave me cancer, forget it," I tell her. "If you're telling me the French gave me cancer, forget that too. I know people like to blame them for everything, but that's going a little too far."

I'm also having trouble with Nick.

I call him up after every important talk with a doctor, and every time he greets me the same way:

"What's the good news?" he asks.

When he hears rough news—the possibility of an ugly reconstruction that could go on for months, the possible problems with chemo—he brushes it off.

"The doctor says you have the best kind," he keeps saying. "You've got nothing to worry about. I wish I could exchange my financial problems for your medical problems."

I keep feeling part of this is my fault: after all, I told him the first day we had to be positive. I also know this is his way of keeping me from being overcome by terror. Sometimes it works and he is wonderful.

"I could have a very strange look for a few months," I

tell him one night, when we're getting ready for bed. "Scars, no nipple . . ."

"So what's a few months?" he says. "When it's over, you have a great new pair. Maybe better."

"I thought you liked these," I say.

"I *love* them," he says, "but you know what they say—variety is the spice of life."

But his constant demand that I lead with "good news" is making me feel that he just doesn't want to hear the bad.

"There *is* no good news," I say to him, finally. "This is cancer. I could lose a breast; I could die; I could be spending the summer with sores on my mouth and a hole in my chest. If you want good news, get yourself a twenty-four-year-old California girl—with no health problems."

Another time, I get him together with Herb, who knows Nick from his newspaper days. Herb does not forgive the men who hurt me as easily as I do. He has been mistrustful of Nick since he went off with his old girlfriend in the fall. "Haven't you broken up with him about 5,000 times already," he said after one of our recent reconciliations. "I don't know if my nerves can take too much more of Nick." With the cancer, Herb is trying to be tolerant, but it's an uphill fight. "I'm having trouble getting through to Nick what a rough thing this cancer deal is," I tell Herb one night, when he's lying on the couch. "Why don't you equate it with him losing his styling gel?" says Herb. "That ought to get him where he lives."

Our three-part meeting, consequently, doesn't come to much.

"Could you explain to Nick this is a difficult, life-threatening disease?" I say.

"Nick, what we're looking at here is a difficult, life-threatening disease," Herb says.

"Could you also say I'm scared, especially of general anesthesia?" I say.

"What's to be scared?" says Nick. "You die on the table, you never know what hit you. I keep telling you, it's the best way to go."

"You're just saying that because you're a guy and you don't like to admit fear of dying," I say.

"My mother isn't a guy; she wouldn't be scared," Nick says.

"Your mother is seventy," I tell him.

"Eighty," says Nick. "But she wouldn't be scared if she was forty. If she was twenty, she still wouldn't be scared."

"What is it with Italian guys and their mothers?" Herb says. "Jewish guys insult their mothers and make jokes about them. Say anything to an Italian guy about his mother, and he's ready to get into a fight."

"Why would anyone say anything about my mother?" says Nick. "She's an incredible woman."

I go back to research.

The week before Easter, I go to Roosevelt to pick up my biopsy slides, which I need for the doctors at Sloan-Kettering. They are the most important medical records I have—the only specimens of my cancer—and they'll be critical in determining my treatment.

Roosevelt, when I return, seems even worse than the first time. The street people who had set up housekeeping on Fifty-eighth Street are still there in their sofa and armchairs and seem to have settled in for the long haul: their possessions are about them in garbage bags, the sidewalk is littered with dirty fast-food containers— just what you want to see next to a hospital. They are very nice, though, complimenting me on my hat and waving like we are old friends. I wave back. For all I know, by the time I come back for surgery, they'll be living in the waiting room. Maybe one will have a fellowship, and I'll look up in OR, and he'll be there, assisting.

The pathology department, where I have to pick up

my slides, is on the ground floor, behind a swinging door which opens to a reception desk and then a rat's run of intersecting halls. I am stumbling through them, searching for pathology, when suddenly I am hit by the smell. It is a smell you don't forget when you have been there: sweet and rotting, with an overlay of formaldehyde. I see the sign just as I am on top of it: MORGUE. A door is opening and I feel like I have suddenly split into two people, one of whom is physically turning the other's face away, so she cannot see inside. The corridors are like a maze in a nightmare, and although I don't believe in fate and don't believe in folk stories, I feel this is a precursor: Death has seen my face near the door of the morgue; and if I come back to this hospital for surgery, he will recognize me and think that's where I belong. If I come back to Roosevelt, they will wheel me into surgery and wheel me out to a refrigerated compartment.

I manage to find the pathology department, which is, as one would expect it to be, next door; but I am now so frightened, I am gulping air. A lab technician gives me a three-by-four-inch padded envelope, which she says includes my biopsy slides and the medical report. I sign for them, certain that everything I am feeling is showing on my face, then beat it toward the entrance, looking for a phone. There is an old-fashioned one in a wooden booth.

I duck into it, shutting the door behind me, crying and hiding. Hide from the Angel of Death. I call Herb. The machine answers. I call Nick.

"Oh, Jesus, you almost gave me a heart attack. I thought something had happened. You just got scared," he says.

"But something *did* happen," I want to tell him. "I felt my death foretold." But he is at work, and I am not a crazy person, so we just talk for a while and I leave.

I don't know what to do. On the one hand, I think I should get away from this hospital and this ugly, depressing neighborhood and go to my house and have a nice, hot bath and get sane. On the other hand, I know that when I am not dealing with cancer, I like this neighborhood a lot. It has great food stores and demented, high-energy New York street life and, most important, is full of thrift shops, which I usually don't get to. I once got *Bells Are Ringing* around here for ninety-nine cents. If I stick around and hit the thrift shops and find some great old show tunes, I decide, it will be much more life-affirming than panicking. Also, maybe I'll be able to find a new *Pal Joey*.

Then, walking down Ninth Avenue, I realize what I'm holding in my hand: my cancer. It seems sort of creepy, going shopping with it. If I go to the Forty-sixth

Street Salvation Army, my favorite thrift shop, will they make me check it? I could put it in my bag, but if my purse is snatched, I'll lose it. On the other hand, if somebody sees me carrying an envelope, they could think it holds something valuable and snatch that. It's the most important thing I own—if somebody steals it, what will I do? Put signs on the trees like they do in my neighborhood when somebody loses their cat? "Cancer missing. Last seen in small brown envelope, vic. Ninth Avenue and 55th. Reward—No Questions Asked." Then, if I get it back, the *Daily News* will do a story like they do when a Taiwanese music student forgets his cello in a taxi and somebody returns it. They'll run my picture, clutching my cancer, and I'll have to look grateful and teary-eyed, while all across town cabbies will be pointing at it, making fun. "*Putz*. Lookit this. She's carrying her cancer in her hand, and what does she do? She goes shopping. Just like a woman."

I do go shopping, just to spite them, but it is unsatisfying. I stuff my cancer in my purse so I don't have to check it and make an incredibly bad buy: a pair of navy and white Ferragamo flats a size too large. When you buy shoes you know do not fit, it is time to go home.

When I do, I find the package with my slides is unnerving me: I have a sense of them powerful and glowing, like Kryptonite, sending killer rays around the apartment. I also don't know where to put them. The flowered hat boxes, where I keep my fancy underwear? The drawer with my foreign currency and passport? I'm also still shook up by the morgue. My shrink has said if I need her, call her. I do. She says she has one minute—her group is coming in. "I'm not sure I can do this in a minute," I say, but I try: my sense of a death foretold, the way my father was diagnosed at exactly this season five years ago, and my fear that I will die like my father. "You're not your father," she says. "This is all in your mind. You're doing this to yourself. Snap out of it." Wonderful. I got cancer—excuse me, I *had* cancer—and my shrink turns into Cher in *Moonstruck*. I call up Heidi, who's less pressed for time. She understands why I am upset. It is insensitive and appalling that a hospital would make one pick up records next to the morgue, she says. I feel better. When I get off the phone, I decide I will demystify the cancer pack. I saw it whole, before I knew it was cancer; am I going to let it bother me now just because I know what it is? What kind of a take-charge attitude is that? I open the package: just a one-page lab report and two little slides, with a bit of translucent tissue that is stained a purple-pink. I give it some death-ray visualization, like I have read about in the books. Then I put on *Bells Are Ringing,* remembering as I do that Judy Holliday died young, of cancer. She left her voice, anyway—that gorgeous mixture of bubble and sass—and who can't smile hearing it? In no time at all I am dancing with an invisible partner to "Long before I Knew You," so lost in dreams it takes me a while to notice Judy has dropped in and plopped on the couch.

"So whadidya do with the slides, finally?" she asks.

"I put them in my sock drawer," I tell her.

"Oh, no," she says. "That's the first place they look."

VIII

YOU SEE THE DIFFERENCE BETWEEN SLOAN-KETTERING AND
Roosevelt the moment you walk in Sloan's Upper East
Side residence: money. The reception desk is banked
with pots of white narcissus; the walls are hung with
tasteful prints; I haven't had so many smiling people asking if they could be of assistance since I was in Los Ange-
les. Herb and I have been tense coming here, steeling
ourselves to see emaciated people in wheelchairs. A few
friends had reinforced that fear: I would see terrible
things at a cancer center, they said; it might be so depressing I should consider treatment elsewhere. That advice, to me, was simply bad. If people in very bad shape
had come to a hospital, I reasoned, it was because they
had reached a point where they were desperate for the
best treatment available. The best was what I wanted.
What would be truly depressing would be to know I had
one of the country's top cancer research centers twenty
minutes from my house and had not considered it. I do,
sitting in the bright waiting room with its Oriental rugs
and deep sofas, see a few people in wheelchairs. I also

spot a few women I assume have lost their hair to chemo-therapy. One wears a baseball cap and has short tufts of hair sprouting here and there, around the band. I find the combination of baseball cap and cancer bracing. "Do not go gentle into that good night—tag the sonofabitch out before he gets to second." I also can't get over the chirping receptionists. "This place is like Disneyland, they're so perky," I whisper to Herb. "Cancerland." A pretty nurse, warm and curvy, with shoulder-length blond hair, comes out to get us. "Cancer Hostess," I tell Herb after she takes my history and disappears with my cancer slides. We wait an hour to see Dr. Jeanne Petrek, who is my second-opinion breast surgeon, but I like her the minute I see her. She's a great-looking redhead who wears a Mickey Mouse watch with her white doctor's coat and has a smart, hyper, full-disclosure style. She enters the room with my slides in her hand, holding them as if they were just another report and not the signpost of my possible early demise. Then, briskly as you please, she challenges my greatest-little-cancer-you-can-get diagnosis.

"This looks like medullary, but medullary carcino-mas are very rare," she says. "And this report is ambigu-ous. 'Infiltrating duct medullary type.'"

I can't believe what I'm hearing. Neither can Herb. We exchange a quick, frightened glance. Infiltrating ductal, the most common form of breast cancer, spreads much more quickly than medullary. I have the sinking feeling I had when I was diagnosed. Dr. Petrek doesn't notice. She's picked up a pencil and is tracing the outline of the tumor on the slide, like a teacher who wants to make sure you get the lesson, though the lesson to me is that I may shortly drop dead.

"Cancers are very dense, packed edge to edge, and infiltrating ductal cancers have edges that look like pointy little stars—very irregular, shooting out," she says. "Medullary has a very regular, round outline, like this, see? This looks like medullary, but I'm going to have our own people look at it."

The fear recedes. She's said "looks like medullary" twice; until the lab guys tell us different, I'll keep believing I've got it.

I ask her whether she recommends mastectomy or lumpectomy. She is far less equivocal on the question than Luke—she sees no reason to do a mastectomy. The top medullary man in the country, Dr. Paul Peter Rosen, is at Sloan, she says. He's done a study of hundreds of breast-cancer patients over a twenty-year period, and he believes that medullary is much less likely to recur than other cancers. It is also less likely to be in the lymph nodes. Whether my cancer is medullary or infiltrating ductal, Dr. Petrek believes it is best to save the breast. Given the clean margins surrounding my tumor, I am a perfect candidate for lumpectomy. She also paints a very different picture of breast reconstruction than Dr. Veteran. It can be a very uncomfortable procedure for large-breasted women, she says. Great, I think, dueling doctors. I suppose it's why people get second opinions, but it's not doing a lot for my confidence about the profession. Dentists agree that drilling a tooth will hurt, even if everyone has a different pain threshold. Why aren't these people in agreement over whether sticking an implant under the muscle of my chest will be painful? Dr. Petrek can't supply any new information from my mammograms either. My breasts, like those of many younger women, are very dense, she says, particularly on the upper quadrant where trouble frequently begins. While it seems certain, given the size of my lump, the tumor was there a year ago, Dr. Petrek can see nothing suspicious when she looks at last year's mammograms.

The notion of combining breast reduction with lumpectomy doesn't appeal to her at all. Nor does she care for reduction surgery.

"Breast reduction is a massive operation," she says. "If you were ever to walk in and see it—ugh. What they do is remove a section of tissue from the lower part of the breast. Then, because they have to bring the nipple up higher, they cut the tissue all around it, and the nipple is hanging there, like on a stalk."

She pauses, giving us all time to visualize. I see from Herb's gray-green complexion he's got the picture and may never unbutton anyone's blouse again. Dr. Petrek moves along.

"There's a lot of rearranging of tissue and scarring which could interfere with spotting another tumor on your mammogram. It would take a lot longer to heal than lumpectomy; you might have to put off radiation treatment. Combining reduction with lumpectomy . . . I don't know if you want to be the first."

She wouldn't do it, she says. But she will discuss it with the head of the breast-radiation unit, Dr. Beryl McCormick, at the next department meeting. She also suggests I get in touch with Dr. Susan Love, the most "ardent, zealous" believer in lumpectomy in the country. I like the fact that this doctor is willing to look into the procedure. I am unable, however, to find someone who has combined lumpectomy and reduction. Love's office knows of no one. Still willing to be first, I have a consultation with a second plastic surgeon. He's recommended by an out-of-town specialist I know; Dr. Luke has heard of him as well, saying he has a reputation for fixing other people's mistakes. The doctor also did breast surgery on a friend of mine. She had had silicone implants ten years ago, then developed an infection, and the doctor had removed them and given her a lift. She was pleased with both him and the results, though she remembered a tense moment as they were wheeling her, groggy and sedated, into the operating room. "Now let's see," the surgeon had said, "are you the one who wanted them so little?" For me, the doctor, a robust, sixtyish guy with a congenial Daddy Doc style, suggests making my breasts as small as possible in order to reduce the amount of potentially dangerous breast tissue. I'm apprehensive.

"I've got a certain kind of body," I say. " I don't want to be Wadler the Pear-Shaped Girl. I have broad shoulders; I have a big chest; I have a big ass."

"Hey," he says, "we can work on that, too."

He's joking. I'm pretty sure he's joking.

"What I mean is, I want to keep things in proportion," I say.

Daddy Doc gets serious.

"Listen, you have cancer," he says. "The medical considerations have to come first."

Dr. Veteran had said exactly the same thing. But something puts me off in this doctor's tone. He seems to be suggesting that having had a diagnosis of cancer, I'm not entitled to the same degree of vanity as other women. He is, on the other hand, willing to do the surgery. After talking with him, Dr. Luke, who had originally been opposed to combining lumpectomy and reduction, is willing to do the procedure. In one operation, the two would do a lymph-node dissection, reopen the original wound to check for additional tumors, and reduce the breasts. As soon as I was sufficiently healed, I would have radiation.

I decide I will do it. Then, an hour later, I decide I will not. Then I change my mind again. Then I talk to Ma. She has been an uncharacteristically good listener during this crisis—in her forty-three years of Jewish motherhood I've never known her to be so unopinionated—but five thousand years of genetic baggage is working against her, and now she snaps.

"I know you said news goes out and it doesn't go in, but I'm the mother and I got a right to an opinion," she says. "My opinion is, I don't like this business of first. First is good for the doctor—he gets to write it up and be a big shot. First is good for the hospital—they get money from the government. But how is it good for you? They don't know what they're doing; they never did it before. And if something goes wrong, it's Goodbye, Charlie—you're the one that has to live with it."

I'm a little surprised. This is a woman whose attitude

toward surgery can only be described as sportive. She had acupuncture for leg pain in China, in a room where there were people with needles stuck in their faces and throats, and calls it "a fun experience."

"I thought you were always saying it was good to be a pioneer," I tell her. "What about medical advances and stuff like that?"

"Let somebody else's kid be the pioneer," she says.

I give it a few days, but ultimately I agree. If reduction could result in scarring and a failure to spot recurrent cancers, it's not a good idea. If the cancer turns out to be in the lymph nodes, and reduction puts off immediate treatment, it's not a good idea either. I can't spend months trying to find someone who's had this procedure—there's a disease to beat; I'm up against time. I don't want mastectomy and traditional reconstruction, either. Why assault my body with an implant if there's no medical necessity for mastectomy?

That leaves me with deciding who to go with as my surgeon. I like both Luke and Petrek. Herb has gone to the library and checked their credentials, and they're neck and neck; they've both taken a lot of time to answer my questions. I feel, however, Petrek may be a bit more forthcoming. I also want the resources of a cancer research center behind me. Luke has had three medullary patients. Rosen has done a study of more than 700 breast-cancer patients, about 5 percent of whom were medullary. I know that a good doctor tries to stay on top of the research, but no one has time to read everything. I've worked in newspaper city rooms; I remember how much information you pick up just being around other people. At a cancer research center, with department meetings and visiting specialists, it's bound to be the same way. If I can't have a cancer contractor, I want a place where all my records and doctors are under one roof. I have that at Sloan. I set the date for surgery with Petrek, for the second week in April—three weeks from the day I was diagnosed. I also ask her if she can give me some positive statistics on survival if the cancer turns out to be in the lymph nodes. She says that finding cancer in the nodes is not uncommon—it occurs in slightly less than half of breast-cancer patients. One of those was Betty Ford. She was diagnosed in 1974, with cancer in two nodes. She is doing just fine.

She also has some good news about my biopsy slides: As is policy at Sloan, two doctors have reviewed them under the microscope. They both say it's a medullary carcinoma.

IX

I DON'T SPEND PASSOVER WITH MY FAMILY. MY MOTHER, WHO made plans to close the Florida house the hour I told her it was cancer, is getting ready to drive north; I don't want to be with the clan in the Catskills. My Aunt Shirley hosts that one, and I haven't told Shirley the full story, because I think she Can't Take It. If I go home, I'm afraid we'll hit the next step in the Wadler serious-illness disinformation campaign: Shirley will Figure It Out.

There are, actually, quite a few people I haven't told: Bernard, who has spent three years telling me secrets he didn't tell his psychiatrists, trusting me to write his true story; my friends Vic and Roberta, who lost a close friend to breast cancer less than six months ago; my friend John, in Paris, whose wife died of the disease.

I end up, then, spending the holidays with Nick and his family. It works out nicely. Easter falls on the same weekend as Passover, and I like Nick's family a lot, particularly his mother. She hugged me the first time she met me. She is big and soft and cushiony. She speaks with such a heavy Italian accent that I sometimes cannot understand what she is saying, which, combined with the old-country thing, makes me feel like I am back with my grandmother. "Iiiii, *maron!*" Mrs. Di Stefano says, when she gets fed up. "What's this 'maron' your mother is always talking about?" I ask Nick finally. "*Madonna,*" he says, giving it the Italian pronunciation. "Madonna, idiot." Since the death of her husband, Mrs. Di Stefano lives with her children, spending a month here, a month there, with each one. When she stays at Nick's, he moves out of his bedroom into the den and sleeps on a futon on the floor. She arrives with a statue of the Blessed Virgin and six suitcases, one of which holds only medicine, and prays three hours in the morning and two hours at night. She prays for the dead; she prays for the living; she prays for Bush—not because she likes him, but because he's President and she feels she should. When I get cancer, she starts praying for me, too. Between, she knits socks and says what everyone in the family is doing wrong and tells stories about sickness.

"Whata you got, my daughter-in-law got, too," she says, lying on Nick's bed, knitting. "First she gitta one side; they cutta it out. The next year it come to the other side; they cutta it out. A cousin of mine, she got it, too."

"Oh, yeah?" I say. "You pray for her, too?"

Mrs. Di Stefano nods yes.

111

"How'd she do?" I ask.

She does a thing with her head and her shoulder that suggests both the mortal coil and an acceptance of the limitations of prayer.

"*Eehhhh*," she says.

We have a nice holiday. The Di Stefano clan arrives at Nick's; the kitchen is filled with the same industrial-size steel pots I remember from the boarding house; there is the same noise level. Nick's son cooks a special risotto; his mother has prepared eggplant sufficient to feed the state of New Jersey; his sister is tasting the gravy for the lamb, invoking the Di Stefano motto that is so like my family's own. ("What is this? Nobody knows what the hell they're doing.") I've brought a cake, because in the Cats-kills you would no more arrive at a family gathering without something in a box tied with string than arrive without your head, but when I try and help in the kitchen, I am hooted out. "Joyce, get out of there; you'll injure yourself!" the Jewish brother-in-law yells. When we finally sit down at the table, everyone joins hands, and Nick's sister says a prayer. It has to do with family. She gives thanks they are all there.

Easter over and my lymph node surgery a week away, I return to medical concerns. I have a bone scan and liver scan for cancer, both of which come back negative—very good news, which I try to remind myself often. I go to a lawyer and make a will, because if anything happens, I do not want the state determining who gets my money. I sign a living will, sent to me from Sloan, saying that if I suffer brain damage, I do not want to be sustained on life-support equipment. I make an outline of the last few chapters of my spy book, assigning rights to Herb. I have been going to the gym a lot, in order to strengthen my heart and lungs for surgery; now I focus on a psychic attack for my stay: most of the patients I see in hospitals, excepting new mothers, shuffle around like depressed schlubs. Analyzing it, I think I know why: bathrobes. Only Rex Harrison could look good in a bathrobe. Hospital pajamas aren't that great, either, though the floppy drawstring pants have possibilities. Casual clothing, I decide, is what is called for. I pull out a bunch of big, floppy, Hawaiian shirts, flowered tights, and pink sandals. I pack my Walkman and make a selection of show tunes and old rock and roll, so that I can keep my confidence up. I have a presurgical session with the shrink, telling her even if the cancer is in the nodes, I will try to beat this disease, and if not, or something goes wrong on the table, I have an interesting life behind me: I have friends who love me; I got to have two grandmothers; I've been in love in Paris; I drank champagne with a spy at ten in the morning; I wrote a few things I liked; I have my friendship with Herb. I had really wanted to stand with someone under a wedding canopy; it would have been nice to live for a few years in France—but maybe it is silly to think you can have everything.

"You have a good life *ahead* of you," she says. "And if you need me, you call me and I'll come to the hospital. We've been together a long time."

The big decision is who to take with me to the hospital. Though my mother is now in striking range in the Catskills, I do not want her with me the day of surgery. Part of this is superstition again: every time my father went into surgery, the family gathered around him, and I do not want Death or his messenger service, seeing a bunch of Wadlers around a hospital bed, to think there's another one, waiting for pickup. Another reason—the stronger one—is that I may be frightened, and if my mother is there, I will have to pretend I am not, so that she won't feel worse.

I don't want to ask Nick to be there, either. The closer I get to surgery, the sooner I learn whether or not the cancer is in the nodes, the more I want to be held; and Nick has made it very clear that illness or no, I am not the woman of his dreams. At night, even after making love, he still puts on a video of *Rope* and uses it to fall asleep, his face as frozen and angry as that of a little boy who feels he has been denied and always will be. I know this look because for most of my life, I have been Nick Di Stefano's psychological twin—discarding the lovers who wanted me, idealizing the ones who did not—but it's a crazy way of life, and I don't want it anymore because now I value time. "Why don't you turn off the movie and try to fall asleep with me?" I say to Nick, meaning, "The best movie is here, right under your nose. It is real and it is me. Love me, you jerk, because now is a gift, and I don't know what I am looking at and soon I could be gone."

It is, part of me understands, a ridiculous hope. If Nick did not value me before, why should he now? Nowhere in the literature does it say cancer will make a person love you.

Anyway, I cannot break through the wall. One evening Nick is so cold, turning his back to me and staring at the television, that though it is one-thirty in the morning, I get up and go home. If you're going to be lonely, I think, you might as well be alone—at least you don't have the extra pain of someone ignoring you. I think of a line from *The Yellow Gardenia,* a novel about the newspaper business, of which I am very fond. "It's too bad you have no mother," a gypsy tells the hero. "You could be rich as cream, but your heart is a beggar without a mother." This is how I feel with Nick: that my heart is a beggar. And yet here I am. In the worst of relationships, I've never been any good at breaking up. When I've tried it with Nick, with whom I had hoped to make a life, it has left me inert with hopelessness. Tackling cancer, even with the terror of death, I do not feel nearly so bad. One night, I talk about it with Herb.

"Have you noticed that I've got this supposedly life-threatening disease, and yet it's easier for me to deal with than breaking up with Nick," I say.

"I never thought about it, but now that you mention it, I think you're right," says Herb. "Why do you think that is?"

"If something goes wrong in a relationship, I think it's all my fault," I say. "With cancer I don't have to blame me. Maybe I should have a T-shirt made up: 'Dating is hard. Cancer is easy.' I could get it for the hospital."

I don't, much as Herb and I always have the urge to go for the gag, order the shirts: there are people dying terrible deaths from cancer; the shirt would be an insult to them. Nor do I rock the boat with Nick by making what he considers to be excessive demands when he ignores me. I have seen posters at Sloan for stress-reduction clinics, so apparently they take the subject seriously; I don't want to risk getting upset by asking Nick to come with me to the hospital—what if he says no? I ask Heidi and Herb to come with me the morning of surgery; Nick will come in the evening, after work; my mother will arrive the next day. Then, the weekend before surgery, I change my mind: Nick is important to me; I want him with me. If Heidi, who has two young children, can arrange her schedule, certainly a fifty-two-year-old bachelor can also. I ask him to come with me. He refuses. "What is this, a test?" he says. I try not to get too upset. I remember the posters at Sloan: Stress Kills.

Mrs. Di Stefano, anyway, is solid. Sickness is her game; when it comes to life-threatening illness, she's the MVP of the Eastern Conference. She knits me a pair of socks and asks what time surgery is scheduled, so she can launch a special prayer. Nick does spend the night before the operation with me. We make love, and that pleases me: if something goes wrong in surgery, my last hours will have been a song, not a whine.

At eight the next morning, as Nick lies sleeping, Heidi and Herb pick me up. We hang out in a room together and, waiting, I am impressed with the sensitivity of the Sloan-Kettering staff. A nurse comes by to see if I have any questions about surgery. When another nurse and an orderly come with a gurney to take me to pre-op and I tell them I would feel very silly being pushed down the hall on a bed, they go into a huddle, bend the rules, and alert pre-op on their walkie-talkie. "Patient walking," they say, and we form a nice little soaring-hospital-costs tableau: a nurse, followed by me, Heidi, and Herb, followed by an orderly and an empty gurney, parading down the hall. Heidi and Herb haven't marched since we protested the Vietnam War; they think it is hilarious I am remaking policy. "Go, Joyce!" they cheer. At the pre-op room, which is adjacent to the operating rooms, I have to tell them goodbye. The room is dimly lit, with a row of eight or nine gurneys and three other patients. I reluctantly climb onto a bed, feeling very scared and alone, knowing there are three other people, feeling exactly the same way, a few feet away. It would be nice, I think, if we could all hold hands, but maybe finally that wouldn't help—we would each still be going in alone. I try to think of a way to handle the fear, because I am supposed to be an adult and not allowed to wail, and find myself, though I am not religious, saying the Shema, the prayer Jews are supposed to say if they are facing death. If God exists and turns out to be a reefer-smoking Be-Bop hipster, I think, I've probably just made another disastrous career decision.

An orderly comes and wheels me into the operating room. Almost everyone is a woman, which gives me a nice, they-all-got-'em-so-they'll-be-extra-careful-of-'em feeling, but I am still frightened of the anesthesia. The more scared I am, the faster I joke. "You know the movie *Coma*?" I say to the anesthesiologist's nurse. "That's my big fear. I have this feeling I'm going to, like, wake up as the featured vegetable in Gristede's next week." I ask her if she can supply statistics, so I can feel better. From the way she rattles them off, I can tell I'm not the first person to ask: twenty years ago the mortality rate from anesthesia was 1 in 20,000 cases; these days it's 1 in 200,000. Then she suggests something else: a sedative called Versed, which will feel like very strong Valium. Next thing I know, I am waking up in the recovery room, slightly nauseated, drifting in and out of consciousness; and then I'm in a hospital room with Heidi and Herb; and soon after that, Nick arrives, with an armful of roses, and the sad, misty look he gets when he is gazing at his son or watching a Disney movie. There's a slight burning, pulling pain near my left armpit when I try to move, and I feel encumbered by tubing: on my right a pouch of a dextrose-and-saline solution is hanging from a metal pole, feeding a clear solution through a needle-thin IV into a vein on the top of my right hand; coming out of my left side, about four inches under my armpit, there's a peculiarly long rope of plastic tubing attached to a plastic pouch. I am so woozy with morphine I cannot raise my head when Nick bends down to kiss me, but I remember the anesthesiologist clearly.

"That lovely woman," I think. "She slipped me a mickey."

I learn later from Dr. Petrek that Versed, the sedative the nurse gave me, has an amnesiac effect. The saline-and-sugar solution is standard for someone coming out of surgery. When an incision is made in the body, it reduces body temperature and causes a loss of fluids, increasing the risk of dehydration and hypothermia. Putting sugar and salt back into the bloodstream keeps all the muscles and tissues working so the body can reheat itself.

I will not know the results of lymph-node dissection for a few days. Until the lab report comes back, Dr. Petrek herself does not know how many lymph nodes she has taken. Lymph fights infection; the nodes in the armpit lie embedded in fat like a cluster of grapes; everyone has a different number. If a patient has a very large or aggressive tumor or if cancer has been found in the blood vessels around the tumor, Dr. Petrek would remove a good deal of tissue, to get as many nodes as possible. As that was not my case, she was not that aggressive. When nodes are removed, lymph continues to collect in that area of the body until, after a few weeks, it finds other channels.

To siphon off the lymph near my left breast, I have all that tubing: a contraption called a Reliavac drain that empties into a transparent plastic canteen. The amount of pale yellow fluid that collects in that canteen is the literal watermark of my release from the hospital. When I get down to fifty ccs over a twenty-four-hour period, they will remove the drain and let me go. I'm cautioned against packing my bags. Big-breasted women, the nurses tell me, tend to throw off a lot of fluid.

Meanwhile, I find the mood on the eighteenth floor, which is known around Sloan as the breast-cancer floor, surprisingly up. After the first day, I have very little pain. I can't raise my left arm directly over my head or touch the middle of my back, but Sloan has daily stretching classes to get the arm back to normal as quickly as possible. My roommate, a research biochemist in her mid-fifties, has had a mastectomy and seems unbothered: maybe she'll have a reconstruction, maybe she won't, she says. There is no guy in her life, but if one comes along, she figures if he's a good man, he'll love her for who she is; if not, the hell with him. My mother comes every day, saying the food in Beth Israel is better and talking for two hours at a clip without paying much attention to anything I have to say, which makes me feel things are back to normal. Nick comes every night, delighted to find a pool table in the sun room but disappointed he can't get up a game. Stéphane, in Paris, sends chocolates. My friends bring magazines and flowers. Every few hours brings another volunteer: a young woman rabbi, which I feel is in keeping with the feminist spirit of the breast-cancer floor; a strolling librarian; a lady who wants to know if I want to learn how to weave baskets. It's proof to me that I really am in a hospital. Where else would anyone believe that what an ailing urban adult really wanted was to learn how to weave a basket?

The volunteer who is most helpful is a former breast-cancer patient the same age as me, who has also had a lumpectomy—somewhere, somebody is doing some careful matching. She's a strikingly pretty woman, in a flowered V-neck dress, and she asks if I understand the next step in my treatment, radiation therapy. When it comes to cancer treatment, I consider myself the smartest kid in the class:

"Takes about fifteen minutes a session; you have five treatments a week, for six weeks," I say. "Some people get tired; the breast can get a little swollen and pink, like you're sunburned. They mark where they're going to radiate you with ink."

"Wrong," she says. "In most places they mark you with ink. At Sloan-Kettering, they give you tattoos."

I stare at her. A tattoo? What's it gonna be? A single-breasted mermaid and SEMPER CARCINOMA on my breast?

"They're very small," she says. "They give you four or five of them. You can have them removed after the treatment, but I think I know of only one person who's bothered," she says. "Can you see mine?"

I look closely at her chest. She has a sprinkling of freckles, like me, and after a minute, I can see one tattoo, about two inches above her cleavage. It's the size of an ink dot. But if someone hadn't explained it to me, and I had just heard the word *tattoo*, I would have been frightened.

There is also a psychological support group. I stay away from it. I still want nothing to do with an affinity group where the common ground is illness. When a social worker comes around, I tell her thanks, but no thanks, too. I'm feeling pretty positive, I tell her. The cancer I had tends not to be aggressive and has a better-than-average prognosis, so though we don't know the results of the lymph-node dissection, I'm feeling pretty positive. If the cancer is in the nodes, I'm going to try to be positive, too.

"You know," she says, "you've used the word *positive* three times now—I get the feeling that's very important to you."

Just like that, it pours out: my concern about stress;

my fear—that I was sure I had rejected—that on some level I contributed to getting this disease. She sighs, as if she's been hearing a lot of this lately.

"There's been a lot of this stuff that's been coming up in the popular literature—people like Bernie Siegel that stress a positive attitude," she says. "We want you to have a positive attitude. As a result of having had surgery you *should* have a positive attitude. But when you're put in a crisis situation and get something like a diagnosis of cancer, it's normal to get depressed and have a lot of negative feeling, a lot of stress. There's not a person alive in the twentieth century who doesn't have stress under normal conditions. To try to deny those feelings when you have cancer just increases the stress and adds an unnecessary burden."

So what about the stress-reduction posters I've seen at Sloan?

"Our approach to illness is to attack everything," she says. "If you feel less stressed, you'll be able to deal with your treatments better, to deal with your family better, to enjoy your life. We're not helping you reduce stress because we feel it can cure cancer. This idea that reducing stress will protect you from further illness—it's like carrying a rabbit's foot: it may make you feel better, because you think you have a solution; but at the same time, you may be setting yourself a goal that is impossible and will only add to your stress. There's a tendency to feel that you have more control than in fact you do—that you can prevent a recurrence with your mental attitude. The problem with that is that it leads to blaming the victim. If something happens, you think it is your fault. The trick to dealing with cancer is to be comfortable with the notion that there are some things we can't control."

Friday, though I'm still throwing off a lot of lymph fluid, they let me go home. I wrap the Reliavac pouch in a red silk scarf and pin it to my sweater and head out with Ma and Herb to a French restaurant in the neighborhood. I have to be very distracted not to enjoy lunch, but I am not in a great mood. I want to get Ma back to the mountains as soon as I can. Dr. Petrek has told me to call her office at three-thirty, and she'll have the report on the lymph nodes. If the news is bad, I won't be able to bear my mother's face. Two-thirty, Herb and I put Ma in a taxi. Three, unable to wait any longer, I call Dr. Petrek. Then I call my brother, who is meeting Ma at the bus station, and Herb, and Nick, and Heidi, and Max.

"They took out twelve nodes," I say. "They're all clean."

X

SCHLEPPING AROUND WITH A SIX-FOOT LENGTH OF TUBE AND a plastic pouch coming out of my side does not make me feel particularly beautiful, but it's not a major problem. I discover that if I stuff the tubing and pouch into a runner's bag around my waist, no one knows it's there. It's more difficult in bed, where I loop up the coils of tubing and pin the pouch to the inside of my T-shirt, but Nick is sweet. "You're embarrassed about this thing," he says. "You know you don't have to be embarrassed with me," and he puts his arms around me, and contented as a kitten, I go to sleep. My left underarm and side are sore; I'm not comfortable sleeping on my left side, but there is no strong pain. Eight days after the surgery, the amount of fluid has gone down enough for Dr. Petrek's nurse, Anne Walsh, to pull the drain. I feel no discomfort when she does—the area around my underarm is numb from the lymph-node surgery and will be for at least a year.

A few days later, notebook in hand, I have my consultation with Dr. Larry Norton, the oncologist who is the chief of breast-cancer medicine at Sloan. I have the feeling, from what other doctors have told me, that in Breast Cancerland, this is akin to being invited to God's for drinks. I wait long enough that it ought to be God—an hour and a half, at which time my medical history is taken not by Norton, but by a young resident, who looks exactly like Doogie Howser, M.D. "These are breasts," I feel I should tell him. "There's one on the left, and if you peek under the shirt, you'll see another one, just like it, on the right. Perhaps you've seen them once in a magazine, sticking way out in front on Madonna. Are you sure you're a doctor?" There's another wait. Then Norton walks in. I feel like Dorothy zipping behind the curtain and spotting the Wizard of Oz: the biggest breast-cancer hotshot in New York is a slight, balding, fortysomething guy in a rumpled white coat and glasses. He's relaxed; he's friendly. Though he doesn't make a lot of jokes, he's got the hip, deadpan style of a comedy writer. He's also got great news for me: he doesn't think I'll need chemotherapy.

"You had twelve nodes taken out; they were all clean," he says. "In 1988, NCI released a study recommending that women who were node negative still have chemotherapy. We follow that, unless the tumor is under one centimeter—that's our cutoff. But there are a few special types of cancers—medullary, papillary, colloid, what's the other one? I can picture what it looks like, but I can't remember its name . . . oh, yeah, tubular—that generally have a much better prognosis than conventional cancers. With these special cancers our cutoff point for chemotherapy is three centimeters. Your tumor was 2.8 centimeters, so we won't be treating you with chemotherapy."

He is ordering an additional test on my original biopsy slides to establish that I did have a true medullary carcinoma, Dr. Norton says. If so, I have every reason to be optimistic. Dr. Rosen, Sloan's expert in breast pathology, has done a study showing that medullary patients whose tumors are less than three centimeters have a better than 90 percent chance of no recurrence.

"Medullary is a bizarre cancer," Norton says. "Most everything about it looks terrible. It has terrible DNA; it's aneuploid, which means an abnormal amount of DNA. That's bad because it means there are errors in the DNA, and that's what makes cancer cells cancer. There's also usually a high S-phase fraction, which indicates a very high rate of growth, which usually means an aggressive cancer. If it weren't for the fact they have lymphocyte infiltration, you would expect them to be very bad cancers, and they can be if they spread to the lymph nodes. . . ."

I like to know everything, but he's getting a little technical for me.

"Lymphocyte infiltration?"

"It means the lymphocytes are infiltrating into the tumor. Lymphocytes are special kinds of white blood cells."

"In other words," I say, "medullary has a higher amount of white blood cells than other cancers?"

"That's it," says Norton. "Medullary is called medullary because it looks like gray brain tissue. The reason it looks gray is because it has all those white blood cells in it."

I remember what my tumor looked like when Luke took it out and have that satisfying little "aha" one gets when a question is answered—"Aha, so that's why that egg-shaped lump was gray." It reminds me of something I've been trying to figure out: how long does Dr. Norton think that tumor was in my body? He says it's hard to know for certain—medullary grows quickly—but he estimates at least three years. As far as spotting any new lumps, Dr. Norton says what Dr. Luke has said: medullary cancers are often missed because they tend not to calcify. For me the problem is compounded because I have cystic breasts.

———

129

"What you have to do is make an effort to de-cyst your breasts," he says. "No caffeine: no coffee, no tea, no chocolate. Give up caffeine as if it's a religion."

I drink no more than a cup and a half of coffee a day, but it's my drug of choice. It jump starts my brain. I can't imagine starting my day without it. Does Norton truly believe my one and a half cups—and my two or three daily Diet Pepsis—affect things?

"I feel a lot of breasts," says Norton. "It's what I do. I've been doing it since the sixties. I'm telling you: you've got caffeine breasts. One cup of coffee a day affects things. Cut out the caffeine, and your breasts will feel much smoother—you'll see the difference."

Norton believes breast cancer *is* on the rise—NCI statistics show it, he says. He personally believes a low-fat diet reduces the risk of breast cancer and recommends it for me. He will also be examining me every six months and doing two blood tests, CEA and CA 15-3, which show the presence of cancer cells in the body.

A blood test that shows the presence of cancer is news to me: if it exists, how come it isn't used at clinics like the Guttman in conjunction with mammograms?

Norton explains that while CEA has been used for several years, CA 15-3 is a new drug that is not widely available. The tests aren't used for screening because they are more effective in spotting metastatic cancer than primary disease: you need tumor bulk and volume to get a reading, and usually primary lesions in the breast are not very large. At 2.8 centimeters I think my tumor *was* very large. Couldn't this blood test have found it, when the mammogram failed? Norton tells me it's unlikely. Metastatic disease is generally ten times the volume of primary disease, and my cancer, large though it seemed to me, was average size. In addition, the blood tests are only from 60 to 80 percent accurate.

The hormone test Dr. Norton orders confirms that I have medullary carcinoma—I won't need chemotherapy.

I am not completely recovered from surgery. I need to nap every day. I still have to go to the hospital two or three days a week, so that the lymph fluid which collects under my arm can be drained. When it collects, I have a swollen, uncomfortable feeling, as if there's a volleyball under my skin. But with the drain removed, and no chemotherapy in my future, I want to celebrate. It's a time I've thought about a lot: A few days after my diagnosis, spotting a pink convertible on Fifth Avenue, I had given Nick a poke in the ribs. "Lookit that. Isn't it great? I love convertibles," I said. "When this is all over, you know what I'd like to do? I'd like to rent a convertible and put the top down and drive to Montauk or go somewhere really wonderful." Only now that the moment is here, it's a dicey call: Nick's money problems are getting worse, and though I am happy to pick up the check for a weekend in Jamaica, Nick is reluctant to accept that. I should have a celebration, he says; he just doesn't feel comfortable letting me cover the expenses. There's never been a time I wanted to dance as much as I do now, and no one I want to dance with more than Nick, but if a weekend in the Caribbean will make him feel bad, I can live without it. We settle on a less extravagant celebration—a night at the Mohonk Mountain House, a rambling Victorian hotel upstate—and I tell Nick I would like it to be my party; when he unloads his money-pit of a co-op, he'll take me away.

I get a bottle of champagne and pick up the rental car, because Nick hasn't bothered to renew his license for fifteen years, and Saturday morning pick him up in front of his apartment. The weekend doesn't get off to a romantic start: Nick is doing the crossword puzzle and, after getting in the car, continues doing it. At the sight of our room, with its mountain view and two double beds, he perks up. We shove the beds together, open the champagne, and don't get to the woods till the next day. And yet, something is off. There is sex, and there is communion, and I have the feeling that Nick is losing himself in the first, not making love to me. When we go walking in the woods, stopping to rest in one of the Adirondack gazebos that circle the lake, I am not altogether surprised to run into Freud. He is on his hands and knees, carving a heart and two names into the bench. "Dependent Loves Narcissist," it says.

"You're telling me I should break up with him, right?" I say.

"Vat?" says Freud. "And miss vatching the two of you in bed? I vouldn't think of it. The *energy* you put into your lost causes."

"You may have noticed, since you've been studying everything so carefully, he doesn't exactly lay there like a lox," I say.

"Exceptional vigor for a man his age," says Freud. "And vhy do ve think that is?"

I don't care what the answer is, I'm mad.

"I know you say there are six people in every bedroom, but you dogging me every place I go with this guy is too much," I say.

"In your case, darling, it's more like *eight* in the bedroom," says Freud. "You also got the editor and the agent. Plus the Vest Coast office of I.C.M. I'm amazed the little *boulevardier* has room to take off his pants."

Nick and I go back to the city. Monday morning, he wakes up and switches on the television next to the bed, without even saying good morning. He lays out his clothes, spending three minutes choosing a tie. He's spent more time choosing a tie, I think, than he has spent with me. Then he moves the television set in front of the bathroom door and disappears into the shower, leaving the curtain partially open so he can watch "Lucy." When he comes out of the bathroom, we fight—a fast fight, left like an open wound, bleeding and unrepaired, because it's Monday morning. Nick goes to work; I go off to Sloan, to see Anne Walsh, the effervescent blond nurse I first thought of as Cancer Hostess, to have a hypodermic stuck in my side. I have no problem with nudity. I like looking at naked bodies on a beach or in a locker room; I don't care if people look at mine. But lately, it's changing. It doesn't matter that aspirating the lymph fluid is painless or that Anne is warm—I'm tired of showing my breast, which is supposed to be a private and special part of my body, to strangers. The smallest pinprick feels like a little assault. Nick's coolness, the continuous resentment about who and what he doesn't have, after I've tried to put together a lovely weekend, feels like an assault, too. It's impossible to find a phone where you have any privacy at Sloan. I wait until I get to the street and then call Nick. The sky is threatening rain. I know I should delay this until the end of the day when Nick gets home, but our fights tear me up; I cannot bear to wait to patch it up. I dial him at the office from an open booth and try to explain.

"It may seem to you like this cancer thing is over, but it's not," I tell him. "My breast hurts; my side hurts; every week I see another doctor. When you flip on 'Lucy' in the morning and freeze me out, it drives me crazy. I just sometimes need to be held."

"Then get yourself another guy," Nick says. "We don't have that kind of relationship."

I don't know what to do—nobody has ever spoken to me so brutally. I feel the old waves of terror that accompany all Nick's implicit threats and, on top of it, a kind of numb outrage. What this man has just said to me is disgusting. He should not be permitted to stay in my life. I should hang up on him. But if I do that, I'll be alone. I answer in a kind of rote.

"I don't care what kind of relationship we have," I say. "I don't think it's an excessive request if a person sometimes needs to be held."

I hang up. As I do, it starts to pour. I have no umbrella, just a light jacket, and in two minutes I am soaked. It's so melodramatic, it's funny. "God must be a soap director," I think. Then I dial Donal, my old boyfriend, finding him easily at the competitor who tore us apart, his photo studio.

"Need a lap," I say.

"Come on over," he says.

He is a big man, with a honey-colored mustache. Except for the fact that he was a newspaper man also, he is the opposite of Nick. His courting style was so shy, so circuitous, that we worked together for a year before I realized that the story tips he was giving me were his way of asking me out. When I finally understood and went to his apartment for tea, it was in such disarray I was shocked. Ten years of *Harvard Magazine* were piled against the living-room wall because Donal was so preoccupied with taking pictures, he never cleaned the house; he had seven cats because he had never gotten around to getting the original pair fixed. They were not great-looking cats, either: a squat, eggplant shaped breed called Vietnamese bobtails, whose ancestors had arrived with a shipment of film at the *New York Times,* as the American press hot-footed out of Vietnam. The cats jumped into Donal's arms one after another to be petted and stroked; every time he put one down, another hairy, blurry trajectory zoomed up and took its place. I had been watching in a kind of a daze, trying to count cats and thus calculate the magnitude of this terrible date; but as I did, I began to notice how patiently Donal petted every cat that leapt in his arms, how gently he put them down. By the time I left his apartment, I was falling in love with Don. Now, soggy and miserable, I arrive at the studio. Donal brews a pot of tea and brings me Humphrey, the fat white studio cat, who eight years ago lived with Donal and me. I love Humphrey, though he makes my nose run. I hold him on my lap, till I sneeze on him one too many times, and Humphrey walks away. Then Donal holds me.

"I know you, I know what you need," says Donal. "You're never going to get it from that man."

"I know that," I say. "It's just these treatments are making me such a baby."

I spend a few days trying to figure out a way to avoid breaking up with Nick, but I can't. The people around me, meanwhile, have had it.

"When a man says something like what Nick said to you, you just have to face the fact that the relationship has become untenable," says the shrink.

"I'm going to come into the city and break his fucking jaw," says my brother Martin.

"No one should be permitted to speak to you like that," says Heidi.

"Maybe you could dump Nick and go out with the mother," says my friend Max.

"If you aren't breaking up with him, *I* am," says Herb.

I call up Nick and break it off.

"Whatever you want," he says, as unconcerned as if somebody he didn't much want to see anyway has just canceled lunch.

When I go to see Anne Walsh next and take off my shirt and bra so she can do the aspiration, I feel so desolate, I start to cry.

"You know, this happens with a lot of women after they have a diagnosis of cancer," she says. "They look at their relationships; they reassess them. A lot of people break up. And then, on top of that, you have the stress of the disease, making everything worse."

She offers to make me an appointment with a Sloan social worker. I decline. I have a shrink, I say. I'm increasing my appointments to twice a week. As for the depression, it's not what she thinks.

"It isn't the cancer," I tell her. "It's me. I've always been lousy with men."

XI

RADIATION THERAPY BEGINS IN MAY, ONE MONTH AFTER SUR-
gery. It strikes me as very sci-fi: First, I have a two-hour
simulation session. Red laser lights shoot down at my
breast as I lie with my left hand behind my head on a table in a dimly lit room, calculating the distance between
radiation machine and breast. Technicians make a plaster
mold of my neck and back, to make certain I am lying in
the same position every time, and take measurements of
my breast, and X rays. They target a rectangle of flesh that
includes my left breast and part of my rib cage and mark
the corners of the rectangle with a felt-tipped pen. Then
they give me five tiny navy-blue pinpoint tattoos. Just as
the volunteer has said, it's like being pricked by a pin.
The only tattoo which might be visible in clothes is the
little dot in the center of my breasts, just above my cleavage. The most interesting part to me is the X rays. After a
six-week radiation treatment to the left breast, I will have
three localized treatments, aimed at the cavity of my tumor in the inner upper quadrant of my breast. In order
for the technicians to find that spot, Dr. Petrek, when she

opened my original biopsy wound, marked the area with stainless steel clips. Looking at my X rays, I see them—a funny little oval of staples, which will be with me for life. It makes me feel a little like a war hero, with shrapnel in my chest. I have two simultaneous desires: I want to go sit on a bar stool, order something in a shot glass, and tell a war story: "Yup, there I was in the shower, buck-naked— always shower naked; embarrasses the hell outta m'boy-friend, but that's the way I am—when I felt this lump. Goddamn thing was as big as a watermelon! . . ." Or I want to go to a store, buy the kind of magnetic Snoopy you put on the refrigerator door, put it on my breast, and see if it will stick.

A few days later, I come back to Sloan to begin the radiation. I have no concerns about the process, but my cancer books say you should bring someone with you your first session; and because of that, and because the breakup with Nick has left me feeling vulnerable and a little shaky, I bring Herb. Just as with surgery, a nurse is waiting to make sure I understand everything. She tells me my breast may become a little swollen and sensitive and may turn pink or even peel, as if I've been sun-burned, and gives me ointment to use three times a day. I'm to protect my breast in the next few months by using a sun-block with a protection factor of at least thirty and wearing a T-shirt. After that, for the rest of my life, I should still protect my breast with a sunscreen at the beach. For my six weeks of treatment I am not to use a deodorant, because most contain aluminum, which can irritate the skin; I am not to swim in chlorinated pools; I should avoid using underwire bras, at least for the left breast. The nurse also has a little Cancer Homemaker's Tip, which it's hard for me to imagine a specialist bothering to discuss: Don't go out and buy a new batch of bras; just remove the wire under the breast that's getting treatment and later stitch it back in.

I am more concerned about internal physical damage. Will the radiation hurt the blood that is moving through my system? Will it kill the healthy cells?

The nurse says blood counts will be done periodically, but that a drop in the white blood cell count is rare in radiation. No damage will be done to my healthy breast cells—they'll regenerate.

Something is not quite adding up here.

"If the cells have to regenerate, they must be getting hurt," I say.

"They're stronger than the cancer cells," she says.

I leave Herb and go into a little changing room, where I take off my shirt and bra and put on a hospital shirt. Then I go into the radiation room. The radiation machine is four feet wide and almost ceiling height, with a long, wide arm jutting out of the top. I get on the table, and a technician slips my plaster form under my head and arm. He spends a few minutes fussing with the angle of my arm until he has it just right. Then he wheels the table back, so I am directly beneath the machine, and shuts the door. I notice, as he does so, it is a very thick door. Outside, he and Herb are watching me through a television monitor. "This is wild," says Herb. "I'm looking right at you." "Oh, yeah," I say. "How do I look?" "Really good," says Herb, "just like Voyeur Vision, on the Naked People channel." I'm not allowed to move, but I can adjust my voice. I take it down two notches, giving Herb a breathy Monroe. "Thank you, Herb," I whisper. "But you didn't come all the way to Sloan-Kettering just to say that. Isn't there something special you'd like to see? Something *she* won't do for you?" "So you watch the Naked People channel?" says Herb.

The technician takes over the speaker. In a moment the mood changes. "We're going to give you two doses of radiation, about a minute and a half each," he says. "You'll hear a little whirring sound, and you'll see a light. Then we'll rotate the machine to the side, and you'll see the light again. Okay?" I'm feeling a little irritated. What is this, the space launch? And yet, with that thick door closed and his disembodied voice and those TV monitors, I'm a little apprehensive, too. I don't know the first thing about radiation; all I know is somebody is going to aim a beam at my chest and kill a bunch of cells—*my* cells. I find myself feeling bad for them. Even if they're cancer, they're living things, too. I close my eyes and silently recite the Shema for them. A whirring sound goes on. I concentrate, trying to feel. Giving it full attention, I can sense the smallest bit of warmth on my breast, like a ray of sunshine coming through a window. The whirring stops, the arm of the radiation machine rotates forty-five degrees, and I'm nuked again. A minute later, the doors open, and Herb and the technician are back. In the changing room I put on my ointment and scrutinize my breast in the mirror—it looks just the same. I also check the clock. Door to door of the changing room, the whole process has taken twelve minutes.

The side effects, as the treatment goes on, are minimal. Within a week my breast does become a little pink and feels very heavy and swollen, as my breasts do before my period, but my skin does not peel. There is one day I get very tired after my first few treatments: going to a street fair with Heidi and her family, I am suddenly so exhausted at two in the afternoon that I go home and go to bed. I have a feeling, however, that is coming from sadness about the breakup with Nick, rather than radiation. I have a little tiredness, as the treatments continue, but not much. Two weeks into radiation I call up *People,* tell them to take me off sick leave, and return to my book. It goes well. My breakup with Nick, however, despite the way women are supposed to reassess their lives after cancer, flounders. Halfway through radiation treatment, feeling life is passing me by on a day the sky is particularly blue, I think of Nick and the beach and call him. The next day, we are at his sister's place on Long Island. We sail and dance to "Red, Hot, and Blue" on the patio, but all through the weekend I am clingy. Nick's sister, who remembers me as a wiseguy reporter, can't quite figure it out. "You sure sit on his lap a lot," she says.

By the end of June my cancer treatment is over. The bills, almost all of which are covered by insurance, total $32,300. There are some things about my experience which bother me, feelings which crop up from time to time which I think of as The Naggers: Why did my gynecologist, who is supposed to be excellent, spend only sixty seconds on each breast whenever she examined me? How come the Guttman clinic, after being concerned enough to have a second doctor look at me, did not aspirate that lump? How come mammograms missed both my malignant tumor and the tumors of my two friends?

I don't like these feelings, because I want to believe doctors have all the answers and American science is the most advanced in the world. I don't like these feelings, because if I was reporting a story and they came up, I would pursue them. I should at least, I think, go back to the Guttman and demand they review my mammograms with me and perhaps review their protocol.

Only now that my treatment is finished, I don't want to pursue it. My friend who had a malignant lump removed four years ago tells me now she never thinks of cancer. This is how I think it should be: over.

It's not that hard to forget, either. I am nervous about lumps and go off to Sloan to have them checked once a month, whenever one seems large or painful. My breast, despite the size of the tumor that was removed, is the same size as the right breast, and looks fine. I learn, now that my treatment is over, that combination breast reduction and lumpectomy *has* been used as a treatment for cancer and the procedure presented to the Northeastern Society of Plastic Surgeons. Late again, I think, though the truth is I'm not deeply disappointed. I see one funny little change in my behavior: as the days grow warm, I find myself wearing very deep cut little dresses to parties. I also realize a deep kinship with the late Lyndon Johnson: I want to show everybody my scar.

Other than that, life returns to normal. Herb and I watch TV and complain about editors. My mother re-ups in the Israeli army, as her way of giving thanks for my health. Before flying off, she comes in to the city and we all go out to dinner, where Ma reminisces with Herb about the motor pool and army life. Ma is much more enthusiastic than Herb.

Nick stops all contact with The Magnificent Obsession, but it does not significantly alter his behavior to me. He goes off alone to a family wedding in Florida over the July 4th weekend, telling me when he returns he missed me and should have taken me—we would have had a great time. "Maybe I'm just one of those guys that has to be away from somebody to appreciate them," he says. He appreciates me for three days. Then he stops. In August, sweating out a 101-degree day, he asks how I'm going to be able to stand his un-air-conditioned apartment when I move in. After the sun goes down, I ask him if this is a serious proposal. He says not really; he just wondered how I would respond. I respond with a right to his chest. I still cannot break it off with him, however; and seeing the hopelessness I continue to have whenever I try, I decide I have to try harder to make a change in myself. I leave my therapist, of whom I am very fond, feeling that if I have put up with a man like Nick for so long, something is not working, and find a new counselor with a more aggressive approach. Perhaps the postcancer life assessment Anne Walsh has talked about is blooming at last: I fought for my life like crazy when I thought I was dying. If I stay with a man who hurts and ignores me, what was the point of my fight? Two months later, I separate from Nick.

In September, I go back to *People*. In October, I am among the 605 Time-Warner staffers to be laid off. My big concern is health insurance: as someone who has had cancer, I know insurance companies will not want to give me a policy or may refuse to cover what they like to call my "preexisting condition." As it turns out, under federal law a company is required to sell an employee their group health insurance for eighteen months. If I then want to convert my coverage to an individual policy, the company cannot refuse. The insurance is expensive—$300 a month—but I can afford it. And though I am nervous about the insecurities of a free-lance life—compounded now by the possibility, however remote, of a recurrence of cancer—I am delighted to be out of *People*. "*Arrivederci* hot tubs," I say to myself. "*Cher*, I no longer care"—and go back to the Village and take off my pearl earrings and finish my book.

For New Year's, in celebration of life, I go to Paris for

the weekend. Bernard, my spy and hero, picks me up at the airport, waving down from the mezzanine with his great, felonious grin. When I get through customs, and he formally kisses me on the cheek, I start to cry.

"I didn't know if I was ever going to see you again," I say.

Though once in a while I see Nick, it is finally over between us. He did, a while back, say, "Enough craziness; let's get rid of the other people and live together already," but it was a mood and it passed. His mother, however, is still praying for me. She is also, Nick says, now praying for Magic Johnson.

XII

THAT WAS WHERE MY CANCER STORY WAS GOING TO END.
Then, nearly a year after the lump has been removed from
my breast, an extraordinary thing happens: my greatest-
little-cancer-in-the-world diagnosis is changed, and I discover that not all of the slides of my original biopsy had
been sent from Roosevelt to Sloan-Kettering.

The discovery comes when, concerned about another sore lump in my breast, I go to Sloan to be examined by Dr. Norton. The lump, Dr. Norton says, is
fibrocystic and nothing about which to be concerned. He
adds, however, that he would like to run some new tests
and asks if I can get my original biopsy slides from Roosevelt—general hospital protocol, after reviewing specimens, is to return them to the institution where a
procedure has been performed. I think nothing of it.
Sloan-Kettering is a cancer research center; I assume they
often have new tests.

I return to Roosevelt and pick up my slides—carefully reading the corridor signs to make sure I don't wind
up at the morgue again. A few days later, after delivering

them to Sloan, I receive a call from Dr. Norton. He tells me they are two *new* slides; unknown to him, the pathologists at Sloan-Kettering had gotten permission from Roosevelt to keep my slides. Based on the slides he had just received, Dr. Norton says, he is thinking of changing my treatment.

"There's an important but subtle distinction between medullary carcinoma and ductal carcinoma with medullary features," he says. "On the basis of the most recent information, we think you're somewhere in between, but close enough to ductal carcinoma that I don't want to take a chance not treating you. After a lot of careful thought and discussion, we want to give you the benefit of a little extra treatment."

His tone is calm, but I know this is serious—he says he'd like me to come in the next day, when he does not normally see patients, so we will have time to talk.

I can't quite believe what I'm hearing. I also have a terrible sense of déjà vu: this whole cancer thing was supposed to be over; is it going to begin again?

I'm also upset that at this late date my diagnosis is being changed: ductal spreads faster than medullary, and if there *are* any cancer cells in my body, for one year they have been having a free ride. I made a point of seeing that my biopsy slides did not get lost—it was why I had gone to Roosevelt Hospital and picked them up myself. I don't understand how any new slides could have suddenly turned up.

Next morning, Herb and I are up at Sloan, sitting across from Dr. Norton, determined to know why my treatment is being changed at this late date. Norton takes it from the top: When my slides first arrived at Sloan-Kettering, two doctors examined them under a microscope. They read "unequivocally" as medullary. One of the little wrinkles about medullary, Norton says, is that while there *are* a lot of white cells, there is an absence of necrosis, or dead white cells. Another thing that distinguishes medullary is its very high rate of cell division, which is called the S-phase division. My S-phase, at 6.5 percent, was lower than average for medullary cancer, but it didn't concern Dr. Norton when he first ran tests a year ago. The slides had tested estrogen negative, which is characteristic of medullary; under the microscope the cells *looked* like medullary. Then on my last visit, my medical records before him, Dr. Norton's eye had gone to the S-phase rate; and for a reason he was not quite sure of, he says, something about it started to trouble him. He pulled the files on Sloan's medullary patients to see how many S-phase rates were as low as mine. None were. Then he got the new slides from Roosevelt. The cells on those slides looked unusual for medullary, there were fewer white cells, and there *was* necrosis. Four pathologists in the breast department had looked at the new slides. It's a close call, but based on the new material, Dr. Norton says, he thinks my cancer is more likely to have been an infiltrating ductal with medullary features than a pure medullary.

I ask how it is possible that Roosevelt did not send all the slides in the first place.

"Hospitals never send over all their slides," Dr. Norton says. "They send a few they feel are diagnostic and keep the rest to cover their ass in case somebody loses them or they don't get them back or somebody sues."

Well, how does he feel about this?

He struggles to be diplomatic.

"I'm not happy, what can I say?" he says. "I don't think there was any malicious intent. I'm not blaming Roosevelt. It's a difficult distinction to make, based on your pathology. Clearly, having more tissue helps you make the distinction. They're supposed to send over slides which are characteristic. . . . I don't know why they chose those two slides."

I'm not happy either. Infiltrating ductal is supposed to be a lot more aggressive than medullary, I tell Norton.

I'm very concerned about having been untreated for a year.

"Your cancer isn't aggressive at all," he says. "You're node negative; the biological characteristics of the tumor are such that it's not aggressive—it's under three centimeters. At its very worst, it's a cancer with a very high cure rate. At its very best, you're looking at a 100 percent cure. You've got somewhere between a good to a fantastic prognosis. Your tumor still might be medullary. It's just that it's got enough in the appearance of infiltrating ductal that I want to give you the benefit of the doubt and have some chemotherapy."

The course of chemotherapy he recommends is CMF—the lower-level chemo treatment the SHARE volunteer long ago described. It's a combination of the anti-cancer drugs Cytoxan, methotrexate, and 5 fluorouracil, as well as two antiemetic drugs—Ativan, which is also a sedative, and dexamethasone, a corticosteroid. The drugs are given in an intravenous drip which takes about forty-five minutes and will be administered once every three weeks, over a six-month period. I'll also have to come in once a week to have a finger-prick blood test to monitor my white blood cell count, which will drop during chemotherapy. I may be more susceptible to infection.

I do not seek a second opinion regarding chemotherapy. The most serious possible side effect is that I may never be able to conceive or may go into early menopause; but at forty-four, with no man in my life, I know my chances of having a baby have already diminished. I am also not as frightened of chemotherapy as some people might be, because I have a very good role model: one of my friends had it and ran four miles a day throughout. She is, it is true, a very disciplined, health-conscious woman—I once saw her order radishes in a French restaurant as a main course—and she may be an exceptional case. From the way other people talk about chemotherapy, I get the idea it's six months of throwing up. I'm a free-lancer. If I can't work for six months, the money stops coming in.

Dr. Norton tells me there's nothing to be concerned about. Nausea, these days, is counteracted with drugs. In the last six months, in fact, a "wonder drug" called Ziphrain has come on the market. It not only quashes nausea, he says, it gets you high. Herb and I can't believe it.

"What's the street value of this drug?" Herb says.

We leave. We still are not certain we have all the answers about this delayed diagnosis. Did Sloan-Kettering mess up by not calling for slides earlier? Is it Roosevelt's error? People Herb and I have told about the slides say the same thing: sue. I don't believe in that. You don't sue someone for making a mistake if they were doing their best; you don't use the courts for dialogue. Anyway, what would be my grounds for a lawsuit? I don't know that any damage has been done. If the cancer goes to my liver, I tell my friends, then maybe I'll sue. Having talked to Norton, I am not that concerned. There is no evidence, from my blood tests, there are cancer cells in me. I view chemotherapy as a sort of head-to-toe mouthwash—something to rinse out the system, to make extra sure any cancer residue is gone. Then, a night or two after seeing Norton, a wave of fear hits. Though it's midnight, I call Herb.

"I just got this terrible feeling that this cancer thing is going to get me after all—that I'm not going to make fifty," I tell him.

"You don't really think that's going to happen, do you?" he says.

I think about it. An American Cancer Society figure comes to mind: the five-year survival rate for localized breast cancer is 90 percent. And that includes all types, not just my maybe-not-the-best-but-still-pretty-terrific-whatever-the-hell-it-is cancer.

"I guess I think I'll be okay," I tell Herb. "I just don't like this eleventh-hour treatment switch."

The last thing I feel like doing, when I'm starting

chemo in four days, is being an investigative reporter, but I want answers: I go to Roosevelt and ask for *all* my slides. Then I ask to speak to the director of St. Luke's–Roosevelt Pathology Department. He's a thin, graying man with an Eastern European accent that seems straight out of Transylvania. And though he's trying—with some effort—to be accommodating, I have the feeling that dealing with patients, rather than their squashy and silent specimens, is not a pleasant change for him. Regarding Sloan's diagnostic switch, he's skeptical.

"I somehow do not believe on account of a little necrosis Sloan-Kettering changes their diagnosis," he says. "What about when the doctor did the aspiration? Have you considered that in the area he put the needle the cells can die and this can result in necrosis? Sloan-Kettering is the leading hospital for cancer therapy; they are always doing tests for every little thing that shows up; maybe with one of their tests, they are finding something. But our slides show: it *is* a medullary cancer."

He is not at all defensive about having sent only two slides—as Dr. Norton had said, it is protocol.

"I sent the key slides I would use to make the diagnosis," he says. "I would never send all the slides—half the time I don't get back the slides I send. If there was disagreement about the diagnosis and the doctor asked to see all the slides, we would send them; but when a patient goes to see a doctor for a second opinion on treatment, we send only the diagnostic slides. You weren't asking for your slides because you were questioning the diagnosis. You were asking for your slides because you wanted a second opinion on treatment."

I can't get over it: This guy sounds like he's more concerned about losing his slides than making sure other doctors see everything. It's like he's the curator of a special collection at the Met—the New York City Breast Cancer Exhibition. Maybe if my book becomes a best-seller, I'll get my own special display stand, next to Betty Rollin and Gloria Steinem. Of course, if either of theirs gets an armed guard, and mine doesn't, I will be very aggravated. I also see a Catch-22: Doctors get all the slides only if they question the diagnosis, but how will they know the diagnosis is questionable if they don't get all the slides? Anyway, I never told Roosevelt that I wanted my slides for a second opinion on treatment and not for diagnosis; I just told them I wanted my slides. Was I supposed to know there was a secret password? That "Give me my slides," which seemed to be perfectly clear, was insufficient? That I had to say, "Give me *all* of my slides"?

I suggest to the doctor that his hospital change its policy and inform other institutions how many slides exist. He says doctors *do know* how many slides exist from notations on the pathology report, that his people only get one or two slides from other institutions, and in the fifteen years he's been at Roosevelt, this is the first time a doctor has changed a diagnosis over their slides. Then he talks some more about how difficult it is to get other hospitals to return his slides.

It all seems crazy to me, but there's nothing I can do. I have two doctors who have looked at the same slides and made different diagnoses. I have been thinking of medicine, I realize, as a science of absolutes. I assumed a doctor would look at a cancer cell and tell you with certainty what it was, just as one looks at the amount of liquid in a measuring cup and gives you a precise count. But breast cancer is apparently not like that; it's more like two coaches disputing a play at a basketball game. I stay with the team with Cancer Research Center on their jerseys.

On a Friday, I begin chemotherapy—Fridays will be good, I figure, because whatever happens, I'll have the weekend to recover. Because Dr. Norton has told me the antiemetics in the chemo mix will make me feel high and dopey and possibly affect my judgment, Herb comes with me, so he can see me home. I also bring my Walkman and a bunch of show tunes to help me feel good when I am having the treatment. *Beauty and the Beast* and *La Cage aux Folles,* I figure, will vanquish anything. The chemo unit is on the seventeenth floor. Most of the dozen or so people in the waiting room look like me—which is to say healthy—but there is one middle-aged woman, apparently an actress, who is so bone-thin it hurts her to sit in a chair. Her family, blond and Connecticut khaki, search the corridors for pillows or a room with a bed; one man, a husband or a brother, tries to distract her with theater gossip from the *Times.* It doesn't work. She whimpers like a three-year-old girl, a drawn-out, high-pitched whine. "It *hurts*," she says. I have a sense of someone in so much pain that inhibitions have fallen away and she has regressed to early childhood, overcome by her needs, unaware of the looks of others. I want to go over, to offer her my Walkman and *La Cage aux Folles,* so she will feel better. But I am afraid that might be intrusive and embarrassing for her and useless. There is also something else: in a worst-case scenario, she is the future I do not want to see. I put the earphones on my head and turn up the volume and look away.

In about an hour, I'm called for treatment. I'm nervous. Though I came to New York in the drugged-out sixties and smoked marijuana in college and still do from time to time, that is as far as it goes. I never had any desire to do LSD or mescaline; drugs that give you hallucinations and make you lose control of your mind are frightening to me. Now Herb and I go to a room with three or four leather recliners, each flanked by a tall metal IV stand. I'm the only patient in the room. The nurse, as always at Sloan, wants me to understand everything: she gives me cards with the names of the chemotherapy drugs and their side effects. I am not, it turns out, getting the new wonder drug. It's mostly used with patients receiving much higher doses of chemo; and since it is a very expensive drug, before prescribing it, doctors want to see if you need it. Nausea, the nurse explains, varies greatly with each person. It is impossible to predict how I will react, but for any nausea I might have in the next two days when the antiemetics in the drip wear off, I am given a prescription for Compazine tablets. The nurse suggests I take it this evening, *before* any nausea sets in.

"You don't want to take the chance that I'll get sick and make the association of nausea with chemo, right?" I say.

"Right," she says.

She tells me that the IV mix, as it is administered, makes some patients chilly, and gives me a blanket. Then she sets up the drip. Each drug, in its own plastic pouch, is suspended from the stand and will feed into a plastic tube, like the estuaries of a river. The nurse puts a little IV needle into a vein on top of my hand and begins releasing the drugs, in order. The first to come down the pipe are the antiemetic sedatives, the steroid, and Ativan. The nurse tells me I may start feeling woozy or drunk. I feel very little, I tell her and Herb—just a little bit woozy. She releases the other drugs into the mix and leaves the room. On my tape deck, the transvestite hero of *La Cage aux Folles* is belting out "I am what I am." The minute the nurse is out of the room, I give Herb a "Let's raise hell" grin. Then I get up, the IV in my hand, and ask him if he'd like to dance. When he declines, I do a nice soft-shoe on my own, using the IV pole, which has wheels, as my partner. "Oh, bartender, no more CMF for the patient in the sneakers and jeans," Herb says. "She's had enough." In the cab I rub up against him. "You know one thing they didn't tell us about this drug? It makes you very affectionate," I tell him. "You think we should take another shot at it? I mean, it's been like a decade." He unlocks my apartment door, steering me into the bedroom. "Say good night, Gracie," he says. I sleep for the rest of the day. Around midnight, feeling sober but tired, I take a Compazine tablet, as directed, so I do not become nauseous. Saturday, though intermittently sleepy, I am well enough to go to the gym. I am surprised and delighted: chemotherapy is a piece of cake. I keep taking the Compazine, just like the directions say, every eight hours. By noon Sunday, I am not so delighted. I feel thick-headed, as if someone has hit me on the head with a sledgehammer wrapped in a towel, but at the same time I'm anxious and speedy. I need to sleep, but when I do, I have terrible nightmares. In one, which I have again and again, I am jumping out my fifteenth-story window. My heart is racing and I am sweating. I find the information cards the nurse has given me—none of my symptoms except the exhaustion is listed, and there is no information card on Compazine. I drag my jumpy, clumsy body to my bookshelves, pull out *The Pill Book* and look up Compazine. I have never seen so many possible side effects: " . . . paranoid reactions, tiredness, lethargy, restlessness, hyperactivity, confusion at night, bizarre dreams, inability to sleep, depression, and euphoria. . . ." I call the doctor who's covering for Norton.

"Jittery, anxious, a feeling like you can't stand still and are going to jump out of your skin?" he says. "Oh, yeah, it's probably the Compazine. A lot of younger people react that way to the drug. Just stop taking it, and next time we'll get you on something else."

At my next chemo treatment, Dr. Norton discontinues the Compazine and gives me a prescription for Ativan. It has none of Compazine's side effects. Two days after each treatment, I am tense and speedy and have trouble sleeping for four or five nights, but after a few sessions I find an Ativan or Valium tablet diminishes that, too.

Midway through the treatment, I also occasionally have hot flashes. They come in the middle of the night, when I wake up hot and sweating, and at first I don't even realize what they are: I think it has something to do with the radiators in my apartment. Then I remember that it's May and the radiators have been turned off, and I realize that the heat is coming from me. A few weeks later my period stops. I know that chemotherapy can result in hot flashes and a disturbance in the menstrual cycle, I know this can also be a sign of menopause, and I don't know what this means. I call up Dr. Norton's nurse. She explains that the drugs which kill cancer cells also suppress the ability of the ovaries to produce estrogen. That triggers the anterior pituitary to produce the chemicals FSH and LH, to stimulate the ovaries. As they are produced, there is a rise in body temperature—hot flashes. Your period can also become irregular. In many cases, when chemotherapy is over, the hot flashes end and the menstrual cycle resumes. It may also resume before then. Or I may go into early menopause. At forty-four that is quite likely. We just have to wait and see.

The other side effects I have been warned about with chemotherapy do not occur. I do not lose any of my hair. I do not develop sores or infections. Except for three days following treatment, I am not tired. I put in a normal workday. I take dancing lessons. I go to the gym three times a week, as I always have. I get winded more easily than in the past, but my body gets stronger—probably because, in order to prove to myself I am not a sick person, I increase my weights.

I also, although I know it is a little loopy, put in a request to Mrs. Di Stefano: I ask she pray that when I am done with chemotherapy, I will have a baby. Herb says this is superstitious nonsense, but I say don't knock it. Who knows what bachelor She-Gods, their own biological clocks thundering, may exist in the heavens, due north of Greenwich Village; and in my experience, Mrs. Di Stefano has been batting a thousand.

XIII

SO THAT IS IT—THAT IS THE STORY OF MY BREASTS AND ME and our cancer. Score: Joyce, One; Cancer, Zero. Or should we say, Score: Joyce, One Trillion; Cancer, Nothing. There are no figures for the worth of a life. I can say with absolute certainty only that I am one lucky guy.

Lucky not just because in the time of the great breast-cancer epidemic mine was so benign; lucky not just for the middle-class privilege that bought me my medical care, but for the terror of the ride. Nothing is real until you are close to it, and for a few weeks I was given something few people have: a dress rehearsal of my mortality. And, while it has not made me a model of mental health, though I remain tempted by the drama and dangers of espionage agents and ladies' men, it changed me. Death, I now see, may not come when I am eighty-five and weary, or after I have solved all my problems or met all my deadlines. It will come whenever it damn well pleases. All I can control—for whatever fight I put up should a cancer make a comeback—is the time between. So when I see something I want, I grab it. If the tulips are particularly yellow, I buy them. If Pavarotti is in town, I make a run to the Met and work the crowd for a scalper. I make time for my friends the way I used to make time for work. If someone treats me disrespectfully, I leave.

As for the mark on my left breast, I am happy to have it. It is the battle scar over my heart; and if no one but my doctor and the girls at the gym have seen it lately, I am certain, believing as I do in musical comedies, that somebody will soon.

"So, how'd ya get that?" he'll ask, our first lazy morning, and I'll say, delighted he has found me, "Glad you asked, 'cause it's a *wonderful* story. . . .'"

Afterword

Susan M. Love, M.D.

JOYCE WADLER HAS WRITTEN *MY BREAST* AS "ONE WOMAN'S Story," but it is a story that has become far too common. It is a story of many women, young and old, gay and straight, poor and well-to-do, black and white. It is a story of an unmarried forty-four-year-old career woman in New York and of a married woman of thirty-five with young kids, living in the Midwest. It is the story of an elderly widow and a young lesbian. This disease strikes all kinds of women indiscriminately, and too often kills them. Why?

Breast cancer is an epidemic. One in nine women will develop breast cancer in her lifetime, and breast cancer is one of the diseases women fear most. Joyce Wadler's story depicts the turmoil women go through when they get this diagnosis; the thirst for information to guide them through the maze of treatment options; the fear they experience facing a potentially life-threatening disease.

Why did Joyce Wadler get breast cancer in the first place? No one in her family had ever had the disease.

Sure, she'd never had children, but that is a very minor risk factor. Actually, most women who get breast cancer have *no* risk factors. The major "risk factor" is simply being female.

Wadler talks about stress. She had been under a lot of stress with her father's death, her career, her relationships—could that have given her this dreaded disease? There are a lot of theories today linking stress to disease, but no evidence whatever that stress causes cancer. On the other hand, stress may affect an already existing cancer. Some studies suggest that high levels of stress decrease the immune system's ability to deal with the cancer. This may be useful to know in terms of making stress-reduction techniques part of your cancer treatment. But it won't affect your chances of getting cancer in the first place.

The sad fact is, we don't know why women get breast cancer. It would be comforting to be able to say, as we can with diseases like lung cancer and heart disease, stop smoking, stop drinking, or cut fatty foods from your diet, and you'll be less likely to get this illness. But we can't do that for breast cancer—not yet anyway.

Why can't breast cancer be prevented, even if we don't know specific causes? What is the magic bullet that will protect us? Perhaps research will provide one. In

1992 the first study looking at prevention was launched. Tamoxifen is an estrogen blocker used to treat breast cancer. In large studies of women with breast cancer it was shown not only to prevent recurrence but also to reduce the incidence of cancer in the woman's opposite breast. This in turn has led the National Cancer Institute and the National Surgical Breast and Bowel Project to set up a study that they hope will determine whether Tamoxifen when given to high-risk women will decrease the risk of subsequent cancer. Sixteen thousand women will participate in this nationwide study. They will be randomized to receive either Tamoxifen or a placebo for the next five years. The hope is that at least sixty-five breast cancers will be prevented in the first five years. This is only a drop in the bucket, but it's a start. In addition, the National Cancer Institute will soon launch a large study looking at whether a low-fat diet can reduce the incidence of breast cancer in post-menopausal women. Both of these studies are important because they represent the first time that federal money is going into trying to prevent this killer.

But they are not enough. We need to look at young women and adolescents and their lifestyles if we are really going to make a dent. What factors in their diets, exercise activity, sleeping habits, etc., may make them more vulnerable to breast cancer in later years. We need to look carefully at the environmental carcinogens that surround us, as well as the hormones used in the beef and chicken which we regularly consume. Maybe it isn't our high-fat diets themselves that are at fault, but the contaminants of the fat. We can't be satisfied with limited research in prevention—the area that is ultimately the most important.

But prevention deals with the future. What about the women with breast cancer today? How can it be discovered early, and how can it best be treated? Joyce Wadler had regular breast exams and mammography. Why wasn't her cancer detected until it was 2.8 centimeters, the size, as she says, of a robin's egg? The concept of early detection isn't quite as straightforward as the public service announcements would have you believe. The implication is that all cancers go through a nice, orderly progression from one millimeter to two millimeters to one centimeter, that you always have an opportunity to find the cancer when it's small and hasn't spread, that potential cure is literally in your hands.

But in reality it isn't that easy. When you feel a cancer, you're not feeling the actual cancer cells. You're feeling the tissue that grows around cancer cells as a reaction to them. And most cancers don't have enough reaction for you to feel until they're fairly large—two centimeters, about the size of a grape. There are unusual cases in which a cancer can be felt when it's the size of a pea. And there are also some tumors that don't incite much reaction and thus aren't palpable until they're quite large, five centimeters or so. The woman with such a tumor will ask herself, "How could this happen? I had mammograms and exams. Is this 'early detection?'" The answer is yes, that she had a sneaky tumor and five centimeters was the earliest it could have been detected.

Another factor in how "early" your cancer is found is the degree of lumpiness or density in your breast. If you have the kind of lumpy or "cystic" (although I dislike that term) breasts Joyce Wadler describes, it may be harder to distinguish the reaction around a tumor until it reaches a moderate size. If you're an older woman with mostly fatty breasts, the tumor may stand out more prominently.

What about breast self-exam? Wouldn't Joyce Wadler have found the lump sooner if she'd done regular self-examinations? Maybe, maybe not. There are no data showing that breast self-exam reduces the mortality rate of breast cancer. Most of us don't do it in a formal way, and we tend to feel guilty that we don't. But most breast tumors are usually found by the woman herself when she isn't particularly looking for anything—often in the shower, as Joyce Wadler did. The basic idea of breast self-exam is that we touch ourselves now and then and have a general sense of how we're built.

Then there's the question of mammography. Joyce Wadler was having regular mammograms, why wasn't her cancer "caught" sooner? Mammograms have the same limits that physical exams have—the cancer needs to have enough reaction around it to be visible. Typically a lump will show up sooner on a mammogram than it will with physical examination—when it's about half a centimeter—but that's still fairly far into the cancer's existence. And the cancer also must be in an area of sufficiently low density for it to show up. This combination of circumstances happens often enough for mammography to be a useful tool, but not a perfect one. Mammography can change the mortality rate of breast cancer in 30 percent of women over fifty years old. That's a lot. But it's only 30 percent. It means that for 70 percent of women over fifty with breast cancer, mammography will not make a life and death difference. Many tumors are so aggressive that cells have spread into the rest of the body even before the cancer can be seen on mammogram, while other tumors are so very slow growing that they will not spread at all. Mammography is less useful in younger women. Their breast tissue is denser and allows for less contrast. It's not clear yet how useful screening mammography is for women between forty and fifty though my own feeling is that it's probably worth it. For women under forty years old, with denser tissue and more vulnerability to risk from radiation, it's more questionable unless a suspicious lump has been found.

It's easy to get lured into a false sense of security with mammography, thinking that a normal mammogram means you're okay. A normal mammogram means you're okay, taking into consideration the limits of the test. I'm not recommending doing away with mammography. It's the best tool we have, so far. But we need to realize it's not perfect. If you have the right kind of cancer in the right kind of breast it can be lifesaving, but anyone with a lump needs to have it biopsied regardless of the mammogram.

The problem is that most cancers have been there a long time by the time we find them. The average cancer has a doubling time of 100 days; it takes 100 days for one cell to double and become two. You need 100 billion cancer cells to have one centimeter of cancer. If you do the math, you'll see that most cancers have been present for eight to ten years by the time you can feel the smallest of lumps. A long time. The tumor gets a blood supply, however, at around year three. This means that cancer cells can be shed into the blood stream very early on, way before we have the ability to detect the tumor. Some of these cells will be killed by the immune system, but others may find their way into other organs, slowly growing and eventually surfacing in a way that is indeed life-threatening.

The size of the tumor is not the only factor that determines whether cells have escaped and, if so, how many. The aggressiveness of the tumor is also very important. This was the basis of some of the recommendations that Joyce Wadler received. Medullary tumors are less aggressive and so less likely to have microscopic cells elsewhere in the body, even when the size is 2.8 centimeters. Some aggressive tumors, on the other hand, will have spread even before the tumor can be felt. Thirty percent of nonpalpable tumors—those only detectable on mammogram—will have spread by the time they are diagnosed. These facts form the basis of the modern approach to breast-cancer treatment.

It would be ideal if we had a blood test or scan that could tell us if any breast-cancer cells had escaped the immune system and were lodged in some other organ. Unfortunately we don't. Therefore we have to use circumstantial evidence to make our best guess. We do scans and X rays to look at the bones, liver, and lungs—

places where breast cancer likes to hide. But these tests are not very sensitive. They show only big chunks of cancer. If they don't show anything we still need to go further—into the lymph nodes. We take out some of the axillary nodes and look at them under a microscope to see if there are breast-cancer cells present. If there are cells it doesn't necessarily mean they are elsewhere in the body, just that there's a higher chance that they are (about 60 percent). If there are no cancer cells in the nodes it doesn't mean you're home free, but rather that there is a lesser chance that there are cancer cells elsewhere (30 percent). We also look at the characteristics of the tumor itself: if it looks aggressive, if cancer cells are seen heading out in the blood vessels or lymphatic vessels, if the DNA tests indicate the tumor cells are dividing a lot, if it is insensitive to hormones.

These are all signs that there might be cancer cells elsewhere. And if, for whichever of these reasons, we think these cells might be there, we treat the woman with some sort of systemic treatment—chemotherapy or hormone treatment. These are forms of drugs that can get into the bloodstream, move into any cells that may be elsewhere in the body, and kill them. This use of adjuvant therapy has been the major change in breast-cancer treatment in the past ten years. And it helps. Chemotherapy improves survival rates by about 30 percent, and in the women it doesn't cure it adds approximately five disease-free years to their lives. Tamoxifen, especially in post-menopausal women, improves survival by about 20 percent, and adds two to three disease-free years to the other women's lives. So when Joyce Wadler's slides were reexamined and it was determined that she did not have the less aggressive medullary tumor, the doctors decided that the size of her original tumor was enough to indicate that chemotherapy was called for.

Chemotherapy isn't automatically given to any woman with breast cancer. Chemotherapy, and even Tamoxifen, have both short- and long-term side effects such as premature menopause, infertility, and, even though rarely, second cancers. So doctors prefer to use them only when the chance of the cancer spreading is sufficient to risk the possible side effects. What we need, of course, is a more precise way of telling who needs systemic therapy and who doesn't, as well as a way of telling if it worked. Researchers are beginning to study this now.

Local treatment is really secondary. This includes mastectomy, with or without reconstruction, or lumpectomy and radiation. Why did Joyce Wadler get two such different opinions? There is no question that lumpectomy/radiation and mastectomy are equivalent in long-term survival of breast cancer. At issue is rather what is the best treatment for any one individual patient. Most women have the same initial reaction as Joyce did: "Get it off!" There is a feeling that your breast has somehow betrayed you and you should punish it by cutting it off. Somewhere in your brain you think that if you can just remove the offending part (and offer it to the gods maybe), you will be able to go on with your life as before.

But the truth is that you can never go back to the way your life was before the diagnosis of cancer. It will irrevocably affect your life. Once the initial shock and "bargaining" have passed, most women respond as Joyce did. They settle in to collect as much information as they can get. Joyce was lucky: her surgeon did not try to rush her. He let her know that she had time to sort things out for herself. This is a most important message: *Breast cancer is not an emergency!* It is very important that you get a second opinion, not only about surgery, but also about chemotherapy, about mammograms, and, as is well illustrated here, about pathology (the interpretation of the slides). It is important that you make the decision that is right for you, and that means a fully informed and fully thought-out decision. Some surgeons will give options and then say, "If you were my wife . . ." But you're not his wife, or daughter or mother or best friend. What's right for another woman may not be right for you. When patients ask me what I would do, I always tell them I don't know. I don't—no one does until they face the situation. And in any case, what I'd do would be based on my own life—my feelings about my body, my feelings about my mother, my particular set of strengths and vulnerabilities and a thousand other factors that have no relation to another woman and what she should do. The choice of local treatment is not a life-and-death decision; by and large, both treatments are equally effective. You can sort it out for yourself.

Joyce Wadler ends her story here, with her treatment nearly completed. But this is where the story for most women really begins. The adjustment to living with what could be a life-threatening diagnosis is enormous, not only for the woman herself but for her family, her children, her significant other. Learning to live with uncertainty is very difficult. Learning to trust your body again when it has betrayed you is very hard. I wish Joyce Wadler good luck in reentering the singles scene, in dealing with her next lover, and in maintaining her insurance in the face of cancer discrimination. I hope she continues to have a strong circle of friends and considers participating in a support group for her own sake and that of others.

The hardest time psychologically is after the treatments are completed.

And I hope Joyce Wadler will join us in political activism to increase funding for breast-cancer research. In 1992, the government's breast-cancer research budget is $133 million. The budget for AIDS is over $1 billion. What this tells us is that political action works. With AIDS, for the first time people with a disease made a difference in the funding and research agenda. I'm not suggesting that money for AIDS research should be shifted over to breast-cancer research, or that some other area of health care or human services be shunted. We don't want a bigger piece of the pie—we want a bigger pie. Our government spends too much money defending the country and not enough defending people's lives. We have been good little girls for too long. It is time for us to start yelling and screaming and being obnoxious. The Breast Cancer Coalition is a new national grass-roots organization dedicated to eradicating breast cancer. We need every woman and man in the country to join with us in saying that this epidemic must stop. We must draw the line at one in nine. We can't let this disease pass on to another generation. Our lives depend on it.